Andrew Smith

A Contribution to South African Materia Medica

Chiefly from Plants in use among the Natives

Andrew Smith

A Contribution to South African Materia Medica
Chiefly from Plants in use among the Natives

ISBN/EAN: 9783337119294

Printed in Europe, USA, Canada, Australia, Japan

Cover: Foto ©ninafisch / pixelio.de

More available books at **www.hansebooks.com**

A CONTRIBUTION

TO

SOUTH AFRICAN MATERIA MEDICA,

CHIEFLY FROM

PLANTS IN USE AMONG THE NATIVES,

BY

ANDREW SMITH of St. CYRUS, M.A.,

AUTHOR OF "SHORT PAPERS CHIEFLY ON SOUTH AFRICAN SUBJECTS."

THIRD EDITION, LARGELY EXTENDED.

J. C. JUTA & Co.: CAPE TOWN; PORT ELIZABETH;
AND JOHANNESBURG.
LOVEDALE: THE PUBLISHING DEPARTMENT.
SOUTH AFRICA.

PRINTED AND PUBLISHED AT LOVEDALE, WHERE BOOKSELLERS WILL
RECEIVE COPIES ON SALE IN THE USUAL MANNER.

PREFACE TO THE THIRD EDITION.

A KNOWLEDGE of the plants imported into the Medical Art is traceable in every country to the early inhabitants, whose experience suggested the maladies in which the medicinal plants they had discovered could be employed with advantage, and whose tentative efforts showed the mode of treating diseases. That applies to this country; but how a drug acts, what it can do, the amount of dose, and with what other drugs it ought to be supplemented or controlled, are things left uncertain. With the plants brought forward here as new to scientific use, much of this has yet to be ascertained by experimentation, and those who experiment are strongly advised to begin with very small doses. Large doses may do great mischief, and they always defeat the object for which they are taken. The plants named here may be classed in a threefold way into —a few important—a number fitted for minor uses—and the rest adduced to show what people resorted to, when they could have recourse to nothing else.

The information that certain plants were employed for given purposes, was procured from many sources; but for the elucidation of the subject, for the opinions expressed, and for other matters generally, I accept the responsibility.

The following acknowledgment is quoted from the Preface to the last Edition: "In acknowledging friendly assistance received in the present enquiry, the first place is due to Professor MacOwan, now Government Botanist, whose aid especially in determining botanical species has always been given in a manner characteristically generous. Among the ladies of the Mission, I have to make very warm acknowledgments to Mrs. Young of Main. As formerly at Lovedale (then Miss Weir), so now she constantly makes use of the medical art as a part of Christian work, and owing to that, and her personal influence, and familiarity with the language, she has access to information from the Kaffir professionals, where others find a sealed book. The value of all her communications is enhanced by the results of her own experiments in the uses of plants. I also owe very cordial thanks to Mrs. Ross of Cunningham for various plants including *Chaetacanthus* an *ubuhlungu*, and Chaenostoma. To the Rev. W. S. Davis of Clarkebury Institution, I have been greatly indebted. The plants *isipetshane* and *imvane*, sent by him, and one of the uses of *inkamamasane* were wholly new to me, besides other things mentioned in the text, but it was of great value to me to find that the results of his enquiries into the properties and uses of various other plants were in harmony with my investigations from quite different sources, chiefly Gaika. His sound judgment and the excellent opportunities he has of experimenting give a value to his conclusions. To C. Birkett Esq., formerly of Fort Beaufort, I owe my first information about the snake-bite plant *Melianthus comosus*, and Kama's use of it, besides other valuable hints. A knowledge of various plants is also due to W. Matthew, Esq., of Eland's Post. Among Native contributors, I will mention but one out of many, Mr. W. W. Gqoba. The moment Mr. Gqoba knew that my object was to bring the use of certain medicinal plants, usually kept secret, within the reach of all men, he placed his own knowledge at my disposal, and did all he could to procure a knowledge of these remedies from others. His intelligence and experience in plant remedies made him an excellent referee. As a Kaffir scholar and for knowledge of Kaffir history and customs he had few equals. One must express great regret at his too early death."

The subject has now been revised and partly re-written, and supplemented by five sheets added to the ten of the former issue, and I have to express very cordial thanks to those who have given aid for this Edition. It happens that they all take a special interest in the medicinal plants of the South African Flora, which gives authority to their statements. The leading only among these communications will be quoted—Rev. Canon H. R. Woodrooffe, M.A., on the *ubuhlungu Crabbea cirsioides*, and its important use; on *Solanum Capense*, and other plants—Rev. Arthur J. Lennard, Principal of Ayliff Institution, on the properties and uses of *Kalmoes* and of *Pelargonium reniforme*—W. G. Bennie Esq., B.A., on the proper mode of using and applying plant remedies, with related subjects—J. F. Soga, Esq.,

Government V.S., on the uses of plants little known, and on Comparative Physiology—W. B. Cumming, Esq., of Tafelberg Hall, on *Withania Somnifera*, and Notes on the uses of numerous plant remedies—Bertrand Niland, Esq., on *Rooi Wortel*, and the use of *Red dagga* in tapeworm—Thomas Van Reenen, Esq., Government Land Surveyor, on a valuable use of *Sutherlandia*, and on *Exomis*—Major Boyes, C.C. and R.M., and Mrs. Boyes, on various things of great importance including the cure of animal blindness. The exact mode of Native treatment for Malignant pustule (Milt-ziekte) was procured for me from Pirie by Miss Margaret B. Ross, of The Grey Hospital. The value of this piece of excellent work could scarcely be over estimated.

As there is a Naturalist of the same name, well known for his Works on South African subjects, an inconvenience is created in publishing anything on the subject of Natural History. To avoid this, I have added for the purpose of distinction the name of a place.

ANDREW SMITH Of St. CYRUS.

October 1895.

CONTENTS.

Chapter		Page
I.	INTRODUCTION	1
II.	COBRA AND VIPER POISONS	10
III.	THE USUAL SOUTH AFRICAN TREATMENT FOR SNAKE BITE—SUGGESTIONS ON THIS TREATMENT	20
IV.	PLANTS USED AS REMEDIES FOR SNAKE-BITE	27
V.	ANTHRAX OR MILT-ZIEK BLOOD POISONING	46
VI.	PLANTS EMPLOYED IN MILT-ZIEK POISONING	55
VII.	PLANTS USED AS TONICS	60
VIII.	PLANTS CONNECTED WITH STOMACH DISORDERS	64
IX.	PLANTS USED IN HEALING WOUNDS AND SORES	72
X.	PLANTS USED IN BLOOD PURIFYING	84
XI.	PLANTS USED FOR SCROFULA	87
XII.	TYPHOID FEVER—RHEUMATIC FEVER—INFLUENZA	92
XIII.	PLANTS FOR COLDS AND COUGHS	97
XIV.	REMEDIES FOR TAPEWORM	104
XV.	PLANTS EMPLOYED IN OPHTHALMIA	110
XVI.	PLANTS USED FOR DIARRHOEA AND DYSENTERY—APERIENTS	114
XVII.	HEADACHE	121
XVIII.	TOOTHACHE—SORE THROAT—EARACHE	123
XIX.	STYPTICS—ITCH—WORMS—EPILEPSY	129
XX.	REMEDIES FOR RINGWORM—KIDNEY DISORDER—LUMBAGO	132

Chapter		Page
XXI.	CANCER	136
XXII.	PLANTS CONNECTED WITH BLOOD-POISONING—Children's &c. medicines—Syphilitic blood-poisoning—Baths—Stitch—A Rash—Bone fracture—Note on slow absorption—On Atropa belladonna	139
XXIII.	LUNG-SICKNESS	151
XXIV.	GALL-SICKNESS — BLACK GALL-SICKNESS — QUARTER EVIL—RED-WATER	154
XXV.	SCANTY MILK—CALVES—DISTEMPER ...	159
XXVI.	BOTS IN HORSES—GLANDERS—SORES—WORMS	161
XXVII.	MISCELLANEOUS	169
XXVIII.	PREPARATIONS FROM PLANTS	184

Appendix

I.	Consumption among civilized natives	188
II.	On Some peculiarities of the African race	195
III.	Fruits in relation to climate	198
IV.	The South African horse-sickness ...	202
V.	The Pasture and the Graminivora ...	205
VI.	A cupping instrument for snake-bite	206
VII.	Strychnine in snake-bite	211
VIII.	Mesembryanthemum tubers as ferments	217
IX.	Snake-poison as a prophylactic—Antivenene ...	218
X.	Mushrooms	223
XI.	Friction	224
XII.	Wounds and Sores	225
XIII.	A respirator or inhaler ...	226
XIV.	Drugs for export	227

A CONTRIBUTION

TO

SOUTH AFRICAN MATERIA MEDICA:

CHIEFLY FROM PLANTS IN USE AMONG THE NATIVES.

CHAPTER I.

INTRODUCTION.

THE Plants described here have most of them been in use among the Natives for medicinal purposes probably for a very long period. Some of them are well known; others are known only to a few, who keep the knowledge of their virtues to themselves with profound secrecy, and occasionally mislead people by showing them some other plant, or by ascribing to a plant some use very different from its real one.

How the virtues of medicinal plants were discovered.—It is at first thought a somewhat difficult question how the native herb-doctors out of the nine thousand flowering plants of South Africa contrived to discover a plant which is a specific for a particular malady. To say it was by accident, or that it was the result of innumerable experiments, and of the experience of ages, is nothing to the purpose, if we consider the doctrine of chances. That was not the method. Any one who has begun to examine plants in order to ascertain their medicinal properties will presently be struck with the fact, that all plants which have medical virtues have a recognizable peculiarity of taste, usually bitter, but otherwise pungent, aromatic, astringent, or acid, and they frequently though not always have a peculiar smell. This enables the observer to throw out the mass of plants, leaving two or three hundred, which is a manageable quantity. Proceeding farther, and setting aside those plants whose virtues are already known, and have been communicated to him by specialists, he experiments on himself to find out the effects of a particular plant, and that presents no great difficulty to those who address themselves to the task, while farther experiments on others will settle the matter. It is easy to see how in this way the use of aloes, of astringents, of tonic bitters, or of appetite-producing plants, was discovered. How they lighted upon the best known plant for curing snake-bite, is not so apparent on this principle, but it seems likely that its narcotic and intoxicating properties in smoking and otherwise were first known, and on being used to deaden pain its more important virtues were discovered afterwards.

Progress would also be made in discovering the specific virtues of plants by proceeding on the very natural idea that plants having similar tastes had analogous properties. This holds true in nature. There is hardly a marked property, which is not shared in more or less by several plants. It is noteworthy in this connection, that two of the chief plants used as antidotes to snake poison have a resemblance in taste and smell,—they are also both Labiatæ—but they are totally unlike in general appearance.

If we suppose then that methods like these are aided by long experience, the results of which are transmitted from one practitioner to another, a knowledge of the virtues of plants, even among a barbarous people, will not appear wonderful.

Scientific use essential.—In making use of plant remedies, it is essential that they should be employed scientifically. Thus the plant called *Geita* or *Nceta* by the Hottentots *(Monsonia ovata)* belonging to the Geranium family has a great repute for curing dysentery and chronic diarrhœa, and yet in many cases it fails, while in others it effects a remarkable cure. These maladies proceed from very different causes, such as from stomach disorder accompanied by acidity, or from a bad liver, or from a congested and irritated state of the colon. In the first two, this remedy which has a sedative property and is mildly astringent, would be of no service. So, the plant called *Birds' brandy (Lantana salviæ-folia)* is an antidote in ophthalmia, and may owe its virtue to its property of killing low forms of life, but if used in cases of inflammation from cold, or for redness of the eyelids connected with nervous dyspepsia and such like, it only does mischief. Its use is in sore eyes caused by poison germs introduced somehow, as for example by flies from putrid matter off the sore backs of sheep, or from infection. It is probable that the loss of repute in many plants is due to trial and failure consequent on an unscientific use. Another common error is to give an overdose, and as medicinal plants are frequently poisonous, the natural result is injury or death.

South African plants of local if not of universal use.—The number of South African plants exported as yet for medical purposes is not great, and whether others may be found worthy to be used in other parts of the world remains to be seen; but there can be little doubt that a mistake has been made in overlooking the use of native plants within the country itself on the notion that if they are not worth exporting, they are of small value here. It is contrary to all analogy to suppose that the country does not produce plants which are antidotes for some at least of its peculiar diseases, especially with so extensive a Flora. Native plants have two advantages over foreign drugs—they can be used fresh— and they are adapted to local forms of disease. The types of disease are not necessarily the same in all parts of the world, and one would suppose that our plants would be an antidote for that form of a disease which is prevalent here. The same principle applies to diseases generally.

Bacteria-killing plants.—The germ theory in zymotic disease is now accepted. But while something has been done to prevent the recurrence of these maladies by inoculation with attenuated forms of the poison-germ, little has been done to find out the means of killing those germs. Quinine is supposed to do so in malaria fever, and carbolic-acid when inhaled those which cause pulmonary consumption. Whether anything come out of it or not, it is at least worthy of attention that many of the plant antidotes of South Africa proceed on the idea of killing poison-germs. The plant used to disinfect meat from an animal which has died of *milt ziekte*, a splenic fever, and various others are of this class, and it is suggestive that one of the chief plants relied on for the cure of snake-bite, ranks also among the antiseptics employed to remedy the effects of eating diseased meat.

Plan adopted in Description.—It is matter of difficulty for non-botanists to identify a Plant especially with so vast a Flora as the South African one. The plan adopted here is to give the Kaffir, Dutch, and English name, besides the Botanical one, and to describe the more obvious characteristics of the plant. The minute botanical characters, and scientific medical terms, have been designedly avoided for the sake of popular use. It must be kept in mind, that the same plant is known by various names among the Kaffirs, Fingoes, and Tembus, and that different plants may be called *i-yeza* or *ubu-hlungu* for the same malady. The description given here is usually exact enough to satisfy a person whether he has got the right plant or not.

How to distinguish Plants of real value.—To distinguish a plant of recognized value from one put forward by some Kaffir empiric on the strength of his own experience, it is of some use to note whether the plant has a well known Kaffir name, which would not be given without some reason. If the plant is called merely *i-yeza* (remedy), or *ubu-hlungu* (antidote) followed by the name of the malady, the value of the indication would depend entirely on whether the name had a wide acceptance or not. There is some danger of using the wrong plant. The Kaffirs generally have some notion of native remedies, in the same fashion as Europeans have of the regular medicines. A knowledge of the really valuable remedies, and how to employ them, is limited to a few, who have an interest in keeping them secret as they make money by them. A sale of these remedies to each other is also common among the Kaffirs.

Only a few important plants.—It would be quite a mistake to suppose that all the Medicinal plants brought forward in this Tractate are plants of high value. Some of them it is hoped will prove of real service in medicine. Others again may be of value because they can be had fresh, or because they are specifics for some malady. In both these classes there may be plants whose most important adaptation will be discovered, when attention is now called to them. Thus the plant *i-nyanja*, used by the witch-doctors as an emetic in their incantations to expel disease, must have been well known for a long period; but its value in lungsickness is matter of recent discovery. After sifting out the plants referred to, there remain a good many of small account medicinally, which yet have an interest as showing what an uncivilized people had recourse to in the absence of anything else, and when the therapeutic action of medicines is better understood, such plants will be objects of scientific curiosity.

Kaffir remedies have a heritage of experience.—Were the plants described in this volume new in every sense and quite untried, the very natural enquiry would be made, what proofs can be given from cases and from experience, that they possess the virtues ascribed to them; but if new to the pharmacopœia, they are not new in another sense. The more valuable plants have been employed by the herb-doctors for ages, and a knowledge of their properties has been transmitted from one to another, so that they have a heritage of experience. No one can understand the value of such an extended trial, who has not in the case of some reputed medicinal plant felt the utter uncertainty what part of the plant to use, how much, for what malady, and whether perseverance in using it is safe, when the symptoms are negative or doubtful. We find, however, the same plant used among the Gaikas, the Gcalekas, the Fingoes, the Tembus, and frequently also the Basutos and Pondos, for the same malady; but not always bearing the same name. This proves conclusively that its use is ancient. The maxim, No cure, no pay—is accepted both by doctor and patient, and that sifts out worthless remedies. The large rewards exacted and readily given for a cure have the same tendency.

Distribution of medicinal plants.—With a Flora so extensive as the South African, there are instances sufficient to establish a somewhat unexpected uniformity or law in the distribution of medicinal plants. One would anticipate that in a country where dryness and humidity form the chief contrasted conditions of plant life, there would be varieties dwarfed from drought, corresponding to the Alpine varieties of Europe stunted from elevation and cold, and so there are to any extent; but besides that, there are frequently two species in the same genus, or two species of different genera, so nearly allied in their medicinal properties that one of them may be substituted for the other, only they do not grow in the same locality. One has its station in moist places or beside rivers; the other is found only in dry ground. In other cases the situation is determined by the soil, whether it is of clay, or sandy, or rocky, while elevation and summer heat also affect distribution.

The Gentians, the Monsonias, and the Agathosmas are examples of this arrangement. Of these there are many species which are adjusted to all the external conditions of soil and climate. So there is a species of Kalmoes, which grows in moist places and beside rivers, and a Berg species on mountains; Leonotis leonurus grows in a clay soil, and L. ovata in rocky places; Acocanthera venenata is plentiful in the Colony, but in the warmer Natal it is replaced by A. spectabilis. Plants for anthrax—Cluytia, Blepharis, Crabbea—are not found in the same localities. Plants for wounds are numerous, but the different species do not grow in the same place.

Those who trace design in multiform nature will see in this arrangement an adaptation for bringing medicinal plants everywhere within reach. Such as look merely for some law will trace the fact just stated to the wider uniformity that some alkaloid, resin, or other principle runs through all the species of a genus, and occurs in a high degree in one or two only, while their situation is fixed by finding conditions of soil and climate, or those conditions evolved them to be specifically what they are. The fact remains whatever view may be taken of its origin.

The principle in question, however, hardly applies to medicinal plants of the highest order, such as cinchona, coca, and the opium poppy, the typical species of which were at first found in one spot, as if to make the different parts of the world mutually dependent.

How to make use of medicinal plants.—Native experience which specifies the plants to employ in various maladies commonly leaves the quantities to use quite uncertain. Those who wish to experiment with medicinal plants are therefore strongly recommended to begin with an extremely small dose. Ten, at most fifteen minims or drops of a preparation, where the root or leaf bears to the solvent the proportion of one to eight, ought to be the maximum dose at first, and should be taken an hour before a meal, and as the real effects of a drug cannot be known at once, it is better on taking one dose to leave the next day blank, and to note the effects on the day after that. If a medicine is likely to benefit, it will then show, and if otherwise, it will with these precautions do little harm. Many of the medicinal plants are poisonous, and in any case large doses are mischievous. To persons in a weak state, they may be extremely dangerous, even if the medicine is suitable. It may happen also that an overdose will produce some secondary disorder in the digestive organs, and the person using the medicine will immediately conclude that it is injurious and throw it up. Care should also be taken to remedy any concomitant derangement of the stomach or bowels, when a plant substance is used as a specific for some malady, else that disorder may defeat the main object.

CHAPTER II.

COBRA AND VIPER POISONS—SIR J. FAYRER ON ANTIDOTES—PLANT REMEDIES HAVE AN AGENCY—SUMMARY OF FAYRER'S CONCLUSIONS—DR. WALL ON THE PHYSIOLOGICAL EFFECTS OF SNAKE-POISONS, AND ON TREATMENT OF SNAKE-BITE.

Two types of snake poison have been recognized, the poison of the Colubrine snakes such as the Cobra, and that of the Vipers of which the Puff-adder is one. Dr. A. Wynter Blyth was the first to isolate a crystalline principle, which is the active ingredient in the poison of the Cobra. He says in his Treatise on Poisons :—" The poison excreted from the salivary glands of the cobra di capello is the most deadly animal fluid known. When first ejected, it is an amber-coloured, rather syrupy, frothy liquid, of feeble acid re-action; it dries rapidly on exposure to air to a yellow film, which readily breaks up into brilliant yellow granules, closely imitating crystals. The yellow powder is very acrid and pungent to the nostrils, and excites a painful (though transitory) inflammation, if applied to the mucous membrane of the eye ; the taste is bitter, and it raises little blisters on the tongue. It is perfectly stable, and preserves its activity for an indefinite time. The dried poison as described is perfectly soluble in water, and if the water is added in proper proportions, the original fluid is without doubt reproduced." p. 455.

"The Viperine poison was examined by Prince Lucien Buonaparte. He separated a gummy varnish, inodorous, glittering, and transparent, which he called *echidnin* or *viperin*; it was a neutral nitrogenous body without taste, it arrested the coagulation of the blood, and injected into animals produced all the effects of the bite of the viper." p. 460.

These two kinds of snake poison are about equally deadly, though they do not act quite in the same manner. When carried inwards by the circulation of the blood, snake-poison by its direct action attacks the great centres of life, causing prostration and death. It also produces the secondary effects of swelling, inflammation, internal ulceration, with others.

The question regarding the efficacy of antidotes in snake-bite is as yet unsettled. Since the publication of Sir Joseph Fayrer's Thanatophidia of India, there has been a disposition on the part of some to accept his conclusion—one which he was apparently anxious to reach, and which he thus expresses:—" To conceive of an antidote, in the true sense of the term, to snake-poison, one must imagine a substance so subtle as to follow, overtake, and neutralize the venom in the blood, or that shall have the power of counteracting and neutralizing the deadly influence it has exerted on the vital force. Such a substance has still to be found, and our present experience of the action of drugs does not lead to hopeful anticipation that we shall find it.

" But I repeat that where the poisonous effects are produced in a minor degree, or when the secondary consequences are to be dealt with, we may do much to aid the natural forces in bringing about recovery. This is not, however, what is meant by an antidote." p. 98.

This definition of an antidote is very exacting, and it does not seem likely that any such antidote will soon be found, either for snake-poison, or for any other poison. The assumption, too, that the known remedies for snake-bite are nothing more than an aid to the natural forces in throwing off the effects of the poison when these are produced in a minor degree, or as dealing only with the secondary consequences, does not agree with the observed effects of administering the best remedies according to South African experience.

In testing the efficacy of a particular remedy there are uncertainties which cannot be got rid of. Supposing the antidote has frequently been used with success in cases of bite from a venomous snake, the poison in these instances may have been exhausted; the bite may have been superficial; or, from some cause only a small quantity of the venom may have been injected. The influence of imagination must also not be left out of account. Confidence in the supposed efficacy of a remedy invigorates the powers of nature, while fear when nothing is done equally weakens them. Occasional failure is another source of uncertainty.

Making allowance, however, for all this, there are considerations to show that certain remedies for snake-bite have a real agency.

1. When the wound becomes livid, when swelling and inflammation supervene, and stings of pain travel from the wound to the nerve-centres, when the pulse becomes small and irregular, and the person becomes drowsy and exhausted, there can be no doubt that the serpent was a venomous one, and that the venom was injected. Very

alarming symptoms frequently occur from fear, but they do not resemble those.

2. When the antidote on being applied externally and administered internally reduces the swelling, puts a stop to the throbs of pain from the wound, as cupping also gradually does, when it removes the sense of exhaustion and creates a feeling of betterness, its remedial action cannot be questioned, nor that it counteracts the direct action of the poison and not its secondary effects merely.

3. When the patient after a partial recovery has a relapse, and is restored by using more of the antidote, this affords additional proof that the antidote is real; and when its use prolongs life for thirty hours when otherwise death would have taken place in half an hour, that also counts for something.

4. Cases of failure to save life are not conclusive against an antidote. The venom being unusually large in quantity, or its being injected into one of the large veins so as to be carried rapidly to the nerve centres, or loss of time, until the mischief is already done, or feeble powers of resistance, may account for the failure.

5. Confidence is supposed by some people to be everything in shaking off the effects of snake-bite. This hypothesis entirely breaks down, as is shown from the case of animals, which are affected by snake-bite exactly like human beings, and are cured by the same remedies; and it does so too in the instance of persons so far gone as to be unconscious or semi-conscious.

6. Plant antidotes have been used with considerable success in South Africa, and the feeling one has about

them is that they are good as far as they go but are not potent enough. Hitherto the preparations from these plants have been of a rude description. They have either been hastily made from the fresh plants by persons who had neither the science nor the appliances of the pharmaceutical chemist to make a concentrated essence for the external application; and who usually have no ammonia. Or, again, they consist of certain preparations made from the bark of the root of *Leonotis leonurus*, or *Red dagga*, sold at extravagant rates, with liquid ammonia as the principal solvent, in which the plant element must undergo disintegration, and in fact it is admitted that these preparations do not keep, and are otherwise imperfect. It is the wish of the writer to make known the chief plants which have been employed in South Africa as antidotes for snake-bite. Medical men and pharmaceutical chemists will then have it in their power to make preparations for themselves, and to employ testing experiments. Some of the plants are valuable. Others are probably of small account, and are given more to show what plants have been resorted to, and on grounds of general interest, than from any supposition of their possessing real value.

A series of highly important experiments on Snake-bite and its antidotes was conducted in India by Sir Joseph Fayrer. A brief summary of some of his conclusions may be given here—" Carbolic acid has a deadly effect on venomous snakes. A few drops put into the mouth of one, and the acid merely touching the head of another, produced convulsions and death in a few minutes. Carbolic acid may therefore be efficaciously used in driving away snakes from cellars and houses.—A venomous snake is not killed by a bite from one of its own species, nor from biting itself; and does not die when bitten by a venomous snake of a different species, as when a Viper is bitten by a Cobra; but innocuous snakes similarly bitten die speedily like other animals.—The injection of ammonia does not arrest the action of the venom; nor does the injection of a solution of strychnia. If snake-poison is mixed with liquid ammonia and then injected, its activity is unimpaired. —The injection of the permanganate of potash solution (Condy's fluid), and the washing of the fang punctures with the same has no effect."

One would imagine, when Sir Joseph Fayrer makes such havoc of the snake-remedies by his formidable experiments, that it would be useless to speak of plant antidotes, but curiously enough he halts just at the critical point. Colonel Showers brought forward a Kelaree, or snakeman, who had succeeded remarkably with his antidote in a number of cases, but who failed when Sir Joseph Fayrer was present, apparently from using an inferior plant, as he could not on that occasion procure the plant on which he relied most, and which he had used in the previous experiments. Sir Joseph reasons, it was the man's own fault if on that critical occasion he did not use his antidote; but his reasoning is sadly out, for he delivers a judgment on what was not before him. The question was not, whether or not the Kelaree was in fault, but whether his antidote was efficacious, or not. The formidable array of experiments given in the Thanatophidia of India goes past the South African treatment of snake-bite; for the methods exploded by these experiments are not such as are practised in this country. The use of plant antidotes therefore remains where it was. These remedies have been followed times without number by the removal of pain and swelling, a sense of relief, the return of strength after prostration, and recovery. It remains to be seen to what limit they can reach, and whether they can be improved. One cannot believe that Nature so bountiful in everything else, has no reply to the bite of serpents.

A series of important experiments was conducted by Dr A. J. Wall under the auspices of the Indian Government, to ascertain the physiological effects of the snake-poisons. His conclusions are, that the poison of the Cobra (Naja tripudians) kills chiefly by producing paralysis of respiration, but it also paralyses the tongue, lips, and larynx—that it is a nerve poison only, with no subsequent blood poisoning, as shown by the fact that recovery was complete when the sypmtoms of the direct action of the poison passed off. It produces extreme salivation, and death is often attended by convulsions which are due to carbonic-acid poisoning.

The poison of the Viper (Daboia Russellii) on the other hand causes directly the most violent conclusions, not followed by death and not caused by carbonic-acid poisoning. The paralysis which succeeds is general, and lasts a very considerable time before respiration is extinguished. The blood becomes incoagulable. The most marked difference is that after the nerve symptoms have passed away the subject has to go through a period of blood-poisoning little, if at all, less dangerous than the primary symptoms. Sanious discharges are also the rule, and albuminuria if the victim live any time.

Dr. Wall mentions as bearing on the causes of the differences of the poisons, that on the duct leading from the poison-gland of the daboia, midway between the gland and its termination at the fang, there is a second gland, completely surrounding the duct, into which it empties.

It does not appear, however, that this contrast between the poison of the naja and that of the daboia applies with exactness to the colubrine and the viperine snake-poisons generally. The venom of the Bungarus fasciatus, a colubrine snake, produces a blood poisoning which takes from two to five days to incubate, and which runs its course like a zymotic disease, producing purulent discharges, and death by exhaustion.

So far as the discoveries of Dr. Wall throw light on the matter, the South African snake-bite remedies appear to be on the right track. Ammonia, a nerve stimulant, though perhaps not merely that, is given internally, as well as applied to the wound. In the Indian experiments and in Australia, it has been injected into a vein, but cannot do any good in that way. The South African snake-bite plants are also some of them powerful antiseptics and fitted to arrest blood-poisoning, and they have also some other properties not yet fully ascertained.

Besides throwing light on the physiological action of the snake-poisons, Dr. Wall has made some important suggestions on the treatment of snake-bite. "For the immediate isolation of the bitten limb, he recommends a strong india-rubber band—such as is used in Esmarch's bandage for bloodless operations—to be bound firmly round the limb several times. This cuts off all possible absorption by preventing circulation, which a tight cord by not fitting itself to the depressions, fails to do, and it secures safety for a surgical operation, till one hour or several hours after the bite. The next thing is to settle whether the patient has been venomously bitten or not. A free incision should be made through the skin at the site of the bite, and the skin reflected back on each side, so as to get a complete view of the subjacent tissue. If no venom had entered, or if the snake was a harmless one, there will be no inflammation; but in the case of a venomous bite there will be intense inflammation in the subcutaneous areolar tissue, not visible from above the skin. In the daboia bite there is a deep-purple patch."*

As the poison is lodged in the tissue underlying the skin, at a depth from the punctures of three to four millimetres, roughly $\frac{1}{8}$ to $\frac{1}{6}$ of an inch, Dr. Wall considers that nothing is effective except the excision of the areolar tissue containing the poison. He says:—"An incision at least an inch and a half long should be made through the site of the bite; the skin should then be excised on each side for three-quarters of an inch. This will freely expose the parts below. The skin should be reflected back in every direction by the scalpel, and with a forceps the whole of the areolar tissue underneath should be thoroughly and completely dissected out, going freely up the limb in the direction of the returning blood current. On the ball of

* Indian Snake Poisons: by A. J. Wall, M.D., p. 136.

the thumb, not only the areolar tissue, but the deep fascia and some of the muscle beneath should be removed, as the fang is capable of sinking in especially deeply here. On the fingers and toes all the tissues should be cut away at the site of the bite till the bone is reached, and if necessary, on the back of the hand or foot, tendon and every structure may be cleared right down to the bone. Life is not to be saved by a haphazard cutting away of anything that comes first, but by an intelligent and careful dissecting away of the part holding the poison, bearing in mind the anatomical peculiarities of each region. . . . . After the whole of the suspected parts have been thoroughly dissected out, the india-rubber band may be removed, but not till then, the part having first been freely washed with a solution of caustic potash or potassic permanganate." (p. 143.) Dr. Wall thinks that suction, burning, igniting gunpowder on the spot, &c., are of little value compared with the careful dissecting out with a knife of all the parts likely to contain the poison. With the more venomous character of Indian snakes, this is no doubt the case; but here in South Africa where they are less venomous, and snake-bite apparently yields in many cases to plant remedies, besides that owing to distances a skilled surgeon cannot be had in time, something else must be thought of. A cupping instrument could not fail to be of value, and could be used by an unskilled person who would not venture to cut and carve with a knife, and might not be certain that the person was poisonously bitten.

CHAPTER III.

THE USUAL SOUTH AFRICAN TREATMENT FOR SNAKE-BITE—
SUGGESTIONS ON TREATMENT FOR SNAKE-BITE.

The usual South African treatment for snake-bite.—The ordinary mode of treating snake-bite in South Africa is to apply at once a ligature, sometimes two, above the bite if in the leg or arm, to prevent the poison from being carried into the circulation. The wound is then encouraged to bleed a little, and among the natives a portion of a horn is sometimes employed in sucking out the venom and the poisoned blood; but though there have occurred such cases, no sane person would suck the wound with his mouth without some suitable tube. Strong suction frequently draws blood from the gums, showing some lesion, and the venom sucked into the mouth might in that way be absorbed into the circulation. Gunpowder is occasionally put into the wound and exploded to remove the poison. After the venom as far as possible is got out in one or other of these ways, the same plant preparation with that used internally is applied to the bitten part, which is sometimes scarified to encourage absorption.

While the wound is being treated, a slight decoction of *Red dagga* (Leonotis leonurus), or of *Klip dagga* (Leonotis ovata), or a hot infusion of *Padde klauw* (Teucrium Africanum), is administered to the patient, and this is repeated afterwards if it is required. A common method of keeping up the patient is to give him brandy or spirits, and that does not produce intoxication, until, as the supposition is, it has neutralized the force of the poison.

This treatment has been partially supplemented by certain Tinctures prepared from the root—especially the inner root-bark—of Red dagga—one of them of a dark green colour, from its leaves apparently, or from Padde klauw—into which liquid ammonia is put and sometimes a little laudanum. They are sold at an exorbitant price, at least twenty times the value of the materials. The application both external and internal is the same as stated.

Defects of this treatment.—There are essential defects both in the Native treatment and in the use of these Tinctures. The common ligatures, even whip cord made as tight as possible, cannot cut off the circulation entirely, as they do not fit themselves to depressions in the bones. Nothing will do so effectively except an indiarubber band wound several times round the arm or leg. Some degree of bleeding, or the explosion of gunpowder, is of little service in removing the poison, which is lodged in the tissues quite beneath all the layers of the skin, and suction with a tube or horn is altogether feeble compared with the powerful suction of a cupping instrument. The radical defects in the Native appliances are the want of a proper nerve stimulant, and the loss of time from not having a plant antidote in readiness. It is just here that these tinctures are of value, as they are ready for instant use, and they contain ammonia a stimulant of some sort. At best, however, they are very defective. The plant extract and the liquid ammonia—which is just water charged with ammoniacal gas—are mixed in the same bottle, and a plant substance will not keep with so much water. The ammonia also tends to escape, which leaves the tincture worthless in comparison with a fresh preparation of the plant antidote. The two ought to be kept in separate phials. The tincture can then have enough of alcohol to preserve the plant extract, and fresh ammonia can easily be had to replace what is weakened, or if it is weak, all the more of it can be used when separate. Still, these tinctures though merely a costly adaptation of a native remedy, have served an important purpose. They have created faith in a particular plant antidote, and they have shown the importance of prompt treatment. With some simple directions they can be made by anyone at the cost of a few pence.

The Natives of the Transvaal have a method of treating snake-bite, which might well be adopted, as it would be supplementary to any other method and would not interfere with it. They dig a pit in the ground and light a fire in it. They then clear out the ashes and spread a skin over this pit, and putting in the person bitten, they cover him up with skins, so as to induce profuse perspiration. After a time, he comes out feeling tolerably well. There can be no reasonable doubt as to the importance of this method, and the relief that would follow, if dense perspiration could be induced. The patient should be covered up with blankets, and bottles of hot water or bags of hot bran should be applied. At the same time hot toddy or tea should be administered. It is assumed, however, that everything has been already done to remove the poison, either by dissecting out the tissues in which it is lodged, or by cupping the bitten spot. Had a little poison been absorbed and gone through the blood, before the ligature was applied, this process would probably remove it.

Suggestions on treatment for snake-bite.—If the species of snake is not known, a venomous bite may be distinguished in this way—the bite of a non-venomous snake merely shows the marks made by a row of small teeth, while the fangs of a venomous snake leave two distinct punctures half an inch apart, and in the tissues below there is an acute inflammation going on, concealed by the skin, but shown by stings of pain. A ligature should at once be applied to prevent the poison from entering the circulation. A flexible indiarubber band or tube wound several times round the arm or leg above the site of the bite is perfectly effective, and will not allow a drop of blood to pass the bandage, as it fits itself to depressions. A soft reim is also suitable, but one must take whatever is at hand so as not to lose a moment. The next thing is, not to scarify, which merely removes surface blood while the poison is lodged deep, but to probe the fang punctures with a lancet or sharp penknife, and apply a cupping instrument to suck out the venom as well as the poisoned blood and lymph. That should be done effectively, for the loss of an ounce or two of blood is a trifle compared with the mischief the poison can do in the blood; and it stands to reason that getting the venom out of the body is of more consequence than all the counteracting agents in the world, since snake poison is a nearly indestructible chemical, quite unaffected by antidotes which merely counterwork its effects. A skilled surgeon might, if it is judged advisable, make an incision in the skin across the site of the bite, display the skin on both sides and cut out the the subcutaneous tissues containing the venom, in the manner Dr. Wall thinks to be indispensable in snake-bite by Indian snakes; but a non-scientfic operator would not care to cut and carve recklessly, and it is for such that a method is described here; for in South Africa, owing to distances, surgical aid would in most cases be fatally too late.

After the effective employment of the cupping instrument, the operator should proceed to the subcutaneous injection of 10 minims, or drops, in bad cases 15 minims of *Liquor strychniae*, procurable from a druggist, by taking up a pinch of the skin between his forefinger and thumb, and inserting the needle of the hypodermic syringe, not vertically downward into the skin, but parallel to its surface, only beneath the true skin, taking care to avoid veins, since injection into them is dangerous, and if it were air, might be fatal. The injection of strychnia should not be begun until the symptoms of poisoning appear in the state of the patient. Strychnia is meant to counteract the paralysing effect of the venom on the motor nerves by exciting them, which would be highly injurious were it not balanced by the opposite effect of the other. Should the first injection not have the effect of counteracting the prostration and coma produced by the snake-poison, it may be repeated after an interval, and even again should they return. A twitching of the facial or other muscles indicates that the limit of safety in employing strychnia, either by injection or internally, has been reached. Along with the external treatment, 10 minims, or drops, of *Liquor strychniae*, described below, should be administered to the patient, and this may be repeated afterwards should his state require it. It is highly necessary to meet the poison from the centre as well as to follow it from near the bitten spot, since the action of the heart may be so weak that absorption from hypodermic injection might be too slow to overtake the action of the poison already absorbed.

To Dr. Müller of Yackandandah in Australia belongs the credit of creating confidence in the use of strychnine in snake-bite, and unquestionably it ought entirely to supersede ammonia as a nerve stimulant. However, like most who are zealous for something new, he flies at any suggestion that strychnine alone is not all sufficient, and scouts the idea that snake venom is in any sense a blood poison. With many snakes it is, and with some it is the chief source of danger. Nothing is more unsafe than to generalize from three or four species of snakes, and to suppose that what holds true of them will apply to the snakes of other countries of entirely different species. Strychnine is a poor antiseptic, and in adopting it as an effective nerve stimulant, it would be proper with South African snakes, especially with the puffadder, the berg adder, and the night adder, when the nerve paralysis is subdued, to administer an antiseptic and also apply it to the wound. *Leonotis*, Red and Klip dagga, has been employed here with considerable success, and ten drops of a tincture given internally, with a little of the same put into the fang punctures with a glass syringe, would most probably be of service. It would also be proper not to discontinue the use of ammonia. It has rendered important service in the bite of some at least of the South African snakes, and it is by no means certain that its action is that of a nerve stimulant only.

Liquor strychniae may be procured from a chemist, or it can be prepared by taking 4 grains of the alkaloid strychnia with 6 minims of dilute hydrochloric acid; adding 2 fluid drachms of rectified spirit, and 6 ounces of distilled water. The proportion of strychnia is 1 grain to 120 minims of the solvent, or less than one per cent. *Dilute* hydrochloric acid is one part of the acid to two of water, nearly. It is unnecessary to be more exact as the acid is not always of uniform strength.

An idea has gone abroad that permanganate of potash would be efficacious if injected in snake-bite, as it certainly destroys the venom when mixed with it. It would, however, be quite useless to inject a solution of the permanganate (Condy's fluid) into the wound, as the nascent oxygen which it yields so readily would seize on the animal matter, not on some element in the poison, by the seizure of which the poison were it in a separate form would be disintegrated and destroyed. The wound might be washed with the fluid.

CHAPTER IV.

PLANTS USED AS REMEDIES FOR SNAKE-BITE.

The more important Plants are put first:—

Leonotis leonurus—Wild or Red Dagga—Kaffir, *um-Fincafincane.*

Leonotis ovata—*Klip Dagga.*

Teucrium Africanum—Dutch, *Padde klauw*—Kaffir, an *ubu-Hlungu benyushu.*

Melianthus comosus—Kaffir, *ubu-Hlungu bemamba*—Dutch, a *Kruidje roer mij niet.*

Blepharis Capensis, and *Crabbea cirsioides*—Kaffir, *ubu-Hlungu besigcawu,* or an *ubu-Hlungu.*

Lasiosiphon Meisneri—Kaffir, *isi-Dikili.*

Acocanthera venenata, and *A. Spectabilis*—Bushman's Poison-bush—Kaffir, *in-Tlungunyembe.*

Chaetacanthus Persoonii—Kaffir, an *ubu-Hlungu.*

Parmelia conspersa—Kaffir, *ubu-Hlungu belitye*—a *Lichen.*

Sebaea crassulaefolia—Kaffir, *ili-Bulawa.*

Cissampelos Capensis—Dutch, *Davidjes.*

Xanthoxylon Capense—*Knobwood*—Dutch, *Paarde pruam*—Kaffir, *um-Nungumabele.*

Imantophyllum miniatum, Hook.—an *ubu-Hlungu bemamba.*

Leonotis leonurus—Wild or Red Dagga—Kaffir, *um-Fincafincane.*

An eager curiosity has existed to find out the South African plant used as an antidote for snake-bite, which has acquired a repute. *This is* the plant. It is the one from which European practitioners have made their noted preparations. There is however one preparation which appears to be made from *Teucrium Africanum*. It is of a dark green colour, which is the colour of the tincture of this plant. *Leonotis leonurus* is a tall plant, growing to the height of 4 to 7 feet. Its leaves are oblong, usually about 4 inches long, and $\frac{1}{2}$ an inch to 8 lines wide, serrate but not quite to the base, rather deeply furrowed. The plant may easily be recognized by the numerous whorls on its stem of light-red or orange-coloured flowers. Its smell is strong and peculiar. The Kaffir name *umfincafincane* is taken from the sugar-birds sipping the sweets from the bottom of its long trumpet shaped corolla. Before the mouth of the corolla opens, which it does when the stamens are mature, the nectar is intensely bitter, but at the moment of opening the sweetness is developed. This means that nature does not wish insect marauders who cannot carry the pollen where it is required, to come and rob the nectary. The *Wild Dagga* or *Wild Hemp* is a totally different plant from the common **Dagga** or **Hemp** *(Cannabis;* Kaffir, *umya)* run wild; but it is so named because its leaves are something like those of the hemp plant, and like them they are smoked by the Hottentots, and are extremely powerful to produce intoxication or delirium. Fanciful stories have been propagated about the mode in which this remedy for snake-bite was discovered, but the truth of the matter is, that this is the Fingo remedy, and has been known to the Fingo herb-doctors for ages. The Kaffir remedy, the one on which they place most reliance, is not this plant but *Teucrium Africanum*.

Leonotis ovata—Klip Dagga.

This is another species of the genus. It is found, as its name implies, among stones and rocks, and will be readily recognized as a *Leonotis* from its whorls of light-red or orange-coloured flowers, only it has usually but one or two whorls, duller in colour, and from having the characteristic smell, similar to but not identical with that of the other species. It is distinguished by its leaves which are ovate, crenate, and much resemble those of the nettle. Their full size is 2½ by 2 inches. In both species the stem is quadrangular, and deeply grooved on each side.

Klip Dagga is regarded as superior to *Red* or *Wild Dagga* in medicinal properties; and in using it for snake-bite the leaves are employed, but *Red Dagga* is preferable when the bark of the root is taken, as it has large roots. In *Klip Dagga* the roots are small even in a large plant. It must not be supposed that the two species are identical in their properties, though they have in some things a common use. We never find it so in nature.

There are two kinds of snake-poison—that of the colubrine and that of the viperine snakes—which differ in nature and also in their effects. It is matter of interest to note that the Kaffir doctors recognized the distinction, of which they must have had an imperfect idea. For the bite of the vipers, they recommend the use of *the leaves* of *Klip Dagga*.

Preparation and use.—In making a preparation from these plants for snake-bite, the leaves of *Klip Dagga* and the bark of the root of *Red Dagga* in equal parts should be employed together— or else the leaves, or root-bark alone of either plant. They must be finely divided, and an infusion made by using not much boiling water and keeping it hot. But as there is usually no time to lose, it would be better to make a tincture which will both keep and be always ready. To do this, put one drachm of the dried plant, or two of the fresh, into each fluid oz. of spirits of wine, or brandy, and steep for a day or two. If the liquid part is squeezed out by putting the mixture into a linen bag, the tincture will be strong, and any remaining vegetable matter will be removed by straining through muslin. The advantage of a tincture is, that the alcohol both holds in solution volatile oils and resins as well as alkaloids, and prevents the disintegration and corruption, which an infusion in water undergoes in one or two days. Liquid ammonia added to a water infusion of vegetable matter, will not preserve it, nor if the ammonia itself is charged with vegetable matter, will that keep. Besides, ammonia is not a suitable solvent except for some alkaloids. The tincture and the ammonia should therefore be kept in separate glass-stoppered bottles, and mixed only for immediate use, if mixed at all. A little laudanum may be put into the tincture to deaden the nervous shock, and externally to reduce inflammation; but only a little, from the tendency of a larger dose to produce torpor.

Teucrium Africanum—Dutch, *Padde klauw*—Kaffir, *ubu-Hlungu*, or *ubu-Hlungu benyushu*.

This is a dark green plant, with the larger leaves three-toed, resembling a toad's or frog's foot—hence the name—

with small white Labiate flowers. The middle lobe of the leaf is the longest and largest, but some of the leaves are slightly cut farther, and some are entire. They are of a lighter green beneath. It is the chief plant relied on by the Gcalekas as an antidote to snake-bite. It is also used in Pondoland and among the Tembus. The Kaffirs employ it in cases of bite by a puff-adder.

With small very venomous snakes, *Teucrium* and the *Wild Dagga* are used together. The mode of preparing *Teucrium* is to make an infusion of the leaves, and in Gcaleka use the caution is added not to make it too hot. A tincture can also be made. The mode of using externally and internally is the same as with the *Daggas*.

There is a small variety of *Teucrium*, which the Kaffirs regard as a distinct species and believe it to be stronger. It grows to the height of about six inches, the leaves are simpler, length half an inch, divided from the base into three spread fingers, each lobe only a line broad. The plant is of a much lighter green than the other, and has a profusion of white flowers. An infusion of it is used for ophthalmia.

Though *Teucrium* is not the principal plant for the purpose, it is used for glanders in horses, and it is employed in disinfecting *milt ziek* meat. Its various uses point to its being a germ-killer. It appears, too, to have tonic properties, but all these things will be noticed under the proper heads.

Melianthus comosus, Vahl—Kaffir, *ubu-Hlungu benamba* (corruption in pronunciation for *bemamba*)— Dutch, *a Kruidje roer mij niet*.

A shrub growing to the height of 5 to 6 feet. It has a compound leaf 6 to 7 inches in length, with five pairs of opposite leaflets and a terminal one, making eleven in all. The leaf-stalk is winged between each pair of leaflets, and just below where the wings cease there is occasionally an odd pair of small leaflets. The leaflets when full sized are 2 inches long, and 6 to 8 lines wide, they are serrate, downy above, with deep cut veins running from the midrib at an angle, frequently hoary with a whitish powder, especially along the veins; beneath they are cottony, and of a much lighter green. The flowers are of a light orange red, green beneath, an inch in the greatest length. The petals are minute, and the sepals have a dark-red spot at the base within. The flowers in this species of Melianthus (honey-flower) are frequented by the sugar birds. This is one of the plants which the Dutch call from its unpleasant smell *Kruidje roer mij niet*.

Melianthus comosus is found in quantity on the banks of the Balfour river, the Philipton river, and other streams flowing down from the Katberg; also on the banks of the Ncera beginning above the high road to King William's Town, and near the old dam on the Lovedale side of the Chumie. It is found in other parts of the Colony, and could easily be cultivated. It grows best in loose porous alluvial soil on a river bank. Its roots there attain a large size. This is one of the most notable of the snake-bite plants.

The parts to employ are the bark of the root and the leaves. If the fresh plant can be had, the best mode is to pound, or scrape down 20 grains—or a piece ¾ of an inch each way and ⅛ of an inch thick—of the bark of the root, and administer in a little water. The juice of the leaves, or a leaf-paste should also be repeatedly applied to the wound. This antidote acts *by producing extreme vomiting*, and the substance vomited is said to be foamy. It is necessary to know this in case of a total misconstruction of the symptom. A tincture of the bark of the root and of the leaves will also serve, and it would appear that the virtue of the former though lessened is not lost by its becoming dry. *Melianthus comosus* can be used for the bite of any snake. This plant can also be used to counteract the poison of other venomous creatures such as the *intonjane*, a poisonous caterpillar found at the top of tall grasses, coated over with pieces of grass. The method of using it is that already mentioned.

It has also the repute of being an excellent general medicine, and gently moves all the digestive organs in succession. Ten grains of the bark of the root would serve for that. It also cures gall-sickness in goats.

This root-bark is very poisonous, and fatal cases have occurred from an ignorant use of it. A criminal trial at Queenstown arose out of one of them, and a test experiment was made. On a decoction being administered to a dog, the dog died, and corn steeped in the boiled stuff was given to fowls, and they died.

The virtue of *Melianthus comosus* in snake-bite has been kept very secret, though many persons have had some idea that it possessed medicinal properties. The late Chief Kama was aware of its character, and it is stated that he brought down a root of it from the Orange River and planted it on the bank of the Ncera at a spot to which I was directed. This may very well have been so, but the plant is now in quantity on the Ncera far from the spot, and it is very plentiful at the Katberg. The story goes, that a Kaffir while walking on the road near Middledrift was bitten on the foot by a puff-adder, and went into Kama's house, who gave him a piece of a root to chew and applied another to the wound, after which the Kaffir went on. This was the root. Kama's mode of using it was either to give a piece of the bark of this root to be chewed and swallowed, or to make a decoction of it and administer—at the same time applying externally a paste of the leaves of the plant, Another mode is to scarify the wound and drop into it the juice of the leaves, and drink some of the juice in water. The driver of a kurveyor was bitten by a serpent at the Orange River, and by this treatment was able to continue his journey, though at first on the waggon.

Rev. John Mtila, of the Gaika tribe, missionary in charge of Knapp's Hope, constantly carried with him a portion of the bark of the root of this plant while itinerating in his district, and he has administered it with success in numerous instances. Some of the Gaika herb-doctors also are familiar with the plant, and look upon it as one of the strongest antidotes.

There is a very singular opinion, that *Melianthus Comosus* can be used as a prophylactic to ward off the effects of snake poison. For this purpose they roast the bark of the root, like coffee beans, and put the powder beneath the skin by incisions made in the wrists and ancles. If this really can have any efficacy, it must be from the chemical ingredients in the root producing some change in the blood. Bushmen also swallow snake-poison as a prophylactic against the effects of snake-bite. In the absence of experimental proof either way, every one can take these opinions at what he thinks they are worth. But before any one scouts the thing as irrational, let him first explain why venomous snakes enjoy immunity from the bite of venomous snakes, while harmless snakes are killed.

Blepharis Capensis, and *Crabbea cirsioides*—Kaffir, *ubu-Hlungu besigcawu* (antidote for the tarantula).
(See MILTZIEK POISONING.)

These plants are employed as a remedy for the bite of several snakes including the puff-adder. A decoction of the whole plant is made, and a very small quantity is administered. They are also used as an antidote for the bite of other venomous creatures such as the tarantula. A paste of the whole plant, including the roots, is applied to the bite, and a little of the decoction is taken internally. The same plants are employed in blood-poisoning from *milt-ziek* meat or diseased meat and in toothache. The coarser species of the same genera are also used in horse-sickness.

Lasiosiphon Meisneri—Kaffir, *isi-Dikili*.

The Lasiosiphons form a rather notable group. They have a heath-like appearance, with a tubular corolloid calyx, limb 5-parted. The flowers form a head with an involucre. The roots are very stringy and are used as sinnet. They are very scorching, if chewed, and will burn the tonsils and throat for twenty-four hours. Three species are used medicinally—*L. Meisneri; L. anthylloides;* and *L. linifolius.* The first of these is distinguished by its saffron or dark-orange flowers. Its leaves are $\frac{3}{4}$ inch long, and less than $\frac{1}{8}$ inch wide, hairy at the back. The involucral leaves are $\frac{1}{2}$ inch long. *L. anthylloides* has bright yellow flowers, very downy, sweet-smelling *in the evening.* The leaves are $\frac{3}{4}$ inch long, but $\frac{1}{6}$ inch broad, wider than the former, and the leaves of the involucre are $\frac{3}{4}$ inch long. All the leaves are covered with hairs on the back. In *L. linifolius* the leaves are longer than in either of the others, and are nearly smooth. The flowers are intermediate in colour between the other two, and have no fragrance. *Lasiosiphon Meisneri* is a considerable bush; *L. Linifolius* is the least, is bushy, and rises from 4 to 6 inches above the ground.

Lasiosiphon Meisneri is found in the lower basin of the Kat River, near its entrance into the Fish River. It is also found in various parts of Tembuland. It is also there used as a cure for snake-bite. The dose is from $\frac{1}{2}$ to $\frac{3}{4}$ oz. of the dried root; but some employ both leaves and root. The preparation is by infusion.

I have also heard of *L. Linifolius* being used for snake-bite, but among the Gaika Kaffirs, its use is in sore-throat.

L. Meisneri is employed in cases of karroo fever, and a paste of the leaves for sores.

It is somewhat difficult to say what its action in snake-bite precisely is, whether it is simply a powerful stimulant, almost blistering in its action, and long continued, and whether the same property does not explain the other uses of the plant. If a small fragment is chewed, it is nearly tasteless at first, but its burning quality is presently developed. Great caution must be used as to the quantity administered. It becomes a question whether the roots of these Lasiosiphons might not be employed with advantage in minute doses as a substitute for arsenic (Fowler's solution), or to make a lotion for the throat in place of a solution of lunar caustic. They would be very much safer than either.

Acocanthera venenata, or *Toxicophloea Thunbergii*, Harv.
—*Bushman's*, or *Hottentot's Poison-bush*—
Kaffir, *Intlungunyembe*, or *Ubuhlungu benyoka*.

Acocanthera spectabilis.

The first named plant is used by the natives for the cure of snake-bite, but it has many uses. It is a handsome shrub, found in thickets and preferring deep shade, from 5 to 10 feet in height, usually the former, with a dense cluster of small axillar fragrant flowers, and fruits of a beautiful carmine, with a bloom when ripening, of the colour and size of a purple grape when ripe. The leaves are ovate, dark green, thick and leathery. A small prickle at the tip of the leaf is a good distinctive mark. The leaf-stalks and twigs are reddish. The whole plant is highly poisonous.

To cure snake-bite they scrape down a small piece of a leaf in cold water, and administer this, which acts by producing vomiting. Another way is to grate down a small portion of the root in water, and administer, while at the same time the pounded leaves are applied to swollen portions of the affected parts, avoiding the bite itself. Fifteen grains of the dried leaves is the largest safe dose.

This plant is a very doubtful remedy in snake-bite, and the utility of its external application is very questionable, but there is no question as to its danger. A woman at King William's Town had been treated by Rev. John Brownlee for snake-bite and was recovering, when a Native doctor administered a preparation from this plant, and she died immediately. A woman at Gaga, in Victoria East, was treated for some malady by a Basuto doctor with a decoction of the bark of the root. She died at once. The doctor was brought into Court, and was in a state of great tribulation about the matter. He offered to swallow the medicine himself, as a proof that it was not deadly. He was allowed to go with a warning, as the Solicitor-General did not instruct the Resident Magistrate to proceed with the prosecution.

Another curious use is made of this shrub in Lower Albany. To prevent the bad effects of transferring cattle from the inland pastures to those near the sea, they break down some of the leaves in a pail of water, and give it to the cattle to drink.

Its active principle has been thoroughly examined by Dr. T. R. Fraser, Professor of Materia Medica in Edinburgh University. He finds it to be a poisonous glucoside, closely related to that of a Wanyika (Somaliland) Acocanthera, which he had previously investigated, but unlike it very difficult to crystallize. He explains the action of *Acocantherin* as follows :—" The chief action of *acocantherin* is on the muscle of the heart, whereby the contraction of the muscle is increased. Hence with small quantities the heart's contractions are rendered more powerful and complete especially when the heart is already acting feebly. When, however, the dose is large, the contraction of the muscle becomes so great that it cannot properly relax when it should do so, and accordingly too little blood enters its chambers, until gradually the chambers become obliterated by the powerful continuous contraction of the muscle substance of the heart. A small dose, therefore, increases the pumping power of the heart, but a large dose destroys its pumping capacity by preventing relaxation and the entrance of blood into its chambers, and so of course produces death."

After this lucid explanation there need be no groping in the dark regarding the use of Acocanthera in snake-bite. Probably the better way will be to set it aside and employ strychnia as a preferable nerve stimulant. It is also apparent why the Native experts stumbled on the use of this shrub in snake-bite from finding it to strengthen the feeble action of the heart, and why they insist on the quantity used being small. The fact that *acocantherin* is a glucoside accounts for the curious inconsistency of certain experts who in using the fresh plant prescribe a very small amount, but a much larger quantity in a boiled preparation with other ingredients. Considerable boiling of a glucoside reduces it simply to glucose.

Acocanthera spectabilis, with the same English and Kaffir

names, is found in the forests of Pondoland and Natal, and its use is similar to that of *A. venenata*. Its leaves are not so shining, and longer, but they afford an uncertain mark in determining the species. The most obvious distinction is that its flowers are in racemes, and twice as large with longer lobes, while those of *A. venenata* are axillar and clustered.

Arrow poisons.—One of the really important uses of these shrubs was to employ them in making poisoned arrows. The Bushmen take the wood of the plant, and pound it to a rough powder, which they put into a clay pot and boil for some time, keeping the lid on as the fumes are noxious, but stirring the liquid occasionally. They then take out the wood, and simmer the remainder till it is reduced to a cupful of a glutinous fluid. They then take it to a Euphorbia tree and shed in the fresh juice, and when they are mixed the poison is ready. It is a brownish substance such as you see in a bee-hive. They smear the tip of the arrow with this, and they use no serpent's poison or other substance in addition. In the Transvaal they extract the poison by the same method from the fruit which the shrub produces in much greater abundance there. The poison is more abundant in the seed or stone. The natives there think that to get this poison into the blood is much more dangerous than it is in the stomach. In this it is analogous to snake poison.

It has been suggested that the designed use in Nature of *Acocanthera* which is found in almost every thicket, is to aid man in gaining the mastery over the savage animals.

The deadly quality of this arrow poison seems to depend

on the combination of a poisonous glucoside having an action on the heart, and *euphorbia* juice. A combination somewhat similar is employed elsewhere. Dr. Messer, of H. M. S. Pearl, speaking of a visit to Banks' Islands, says:—
"The plants used in these islands, from which poison for arrows is got, are '*Toe*' a species of Euphorbiaceae, and '*Loke*' a climbing plant allied to Strychnia. The effects are inflammation and occasionally tetanus." Other poisons for arrows are used in South Africa. Livingstone, in describing his journey through to the West Coast, speaks of a grub whose viscera were tied round the arrow point, and Chapman states that between Amraal's country and Lake Ngami, the juices of a kind of beetle furnished a deadly poison. So effective was this that the lions in that region had been exterminated. It is believed that arsenic scraped from the interior of caves, and also the poison of the yellow serpent have been employed for poisoning arrows.

Chaetacanthus Persoonii, T. Anders., or *Calophanes* P.— Kaffir, *ubu-Hlungu*.

This is a herbaceous plant with small rounded leaves, very bitter, with very small yellow flowers, corolla funnel-shaped with 5-parted limb. It is found at Cunningham in Transkei. Like some other Acanthaceous plants it is employed in the cure of snake-bite.

Parmelia conspersa—Kaffir, *Ubu-Lembu belitye*—A lichen.

This is a lichen of a greenish gray found on stones, which cannot be taken off except by scraping. There may be more than one species which will serve the purpose.

The greener it is, the better. When dried up, it is valueless.

This lichen is used for snake-bite, and for the bite of a lizard, *u-Nqinishe* (stump-tail), which the Kaffirs and many Europeans firmly believe to be venomous, while naturalists say it is the *gecko* and harmless. Cases have occurred, where a bite *ascribed to it* has been followed by enormous swelling and other toxic symptoms. There is something yet to be cleared up about the matter. The dose of the lichen is a tablespoonful scraped off and given internally in cold water. If there is a puncture, the lichen is powdered and put into the puncture when scarified. It is said to draw out a humour. The lichen is administered when poisoning is merely suspected. Some Kaffir doctors believe they can dectect poisoning from the bite of a creature suspected to be venomous, from the character of the pulse.

Sebaea crassulaefolia—Kaffir, *ili-Bulawa.*

This belongs to the Order Gentianeae, and has the characteristic bitter taste of gentian. The corolla is bright yellow, with a short tube and a spreading limb of 5 lobes. The sepals of the calyx are keeled, the keel alone being green, the rest whitish. The leaves are sessile, nearly kidney shaped, $\frac{3}{8}$ inch broad, in pairs opposite, each pair at right angles to the next above and below, placed at the joints of the stem which are $\frac{1}{2}$ an inch long, but shortening towards the top, and the stem is four sided almost keeled at the angles. The plant grows among the grass in pastures, and varies in height from 5 to 10 inches, being larger in moist situations.

This *Sebaea*, and several of the other species have similar properties, it is employed in snake-bite, and is alleged to be a specific for the bite of the puff-adder. Among cases mentioned is that of a native boy who was bitten by a puff-adder out in the veldt, and saved himself from serious consequences by chewing the leaves and swallowing the juice, some of which he also applied to the wound. A farmer also has repeatedly employed *Sebaea* with success in cases of cattle and horses bitten by snakes. The dose he gives is half a pint of an infusion made of the whole plant.

It is useless to explain away these cases. Sebaea must have some virtue in puff-adder bite. Perhaps it acts antiseptically to prevent a disintegration of the blood, which is one effect caused by the venom of this snake, and possibly it may be a nerve stimulant in some degree. The plant no doubt has the general properties of the officinal Gentian. It is used by the Kaffirs for *ili-hlaba*, stitch. Perhaps this humble but pretty flower serves a more important purpose in the economy of nature, as is elsewhere suggested.

Cissampelos Capensis—Dutch, *Davidjes.*

As this shrub is well known to the Colonists, and is already described by Dr. Pappe, it is referred to here for the purpose of stating, that it is sometimes employed by Kaffir herb-doctors in snake-bite—a paste of the leaves being applied to the wound, and a decoction of the root given internally. This is not quoted for its real importance, but rather as throwing light on the whole question of remedies for snake-bite.

To the above Plants which I am not aware of being published before in connection with Snake-bite, two others may now be added

Xanthoxylon Capense—Knobwood—D. *Paarde praam*—K. *um-Nungumabele.*

A decoction is made from the root of this tree for snake-bite. (See MILTZIEK POISONING.)

Imantophyllum miniatum, Hook.—K. an *ubu-Hhlungu be-mamba.*

A plant with large strap-shaped leaves and orange-scarlet widely opening flowers, found in St. John's River district and northwards. The rootstock is said to be a cure for the bite of the puff-adder.

Dr. Pappe also mentions the root of *Polygala serpentaria,* E. and Z.—D. *Kaffir Slangenwortel.* I do not happen to have heard of its being used.

The natives of South Africa have saved many lives from the deadly effects of snake-bite by having recourse to plant antidotes on the experimental method, without knowing definitely how they act. An opinion may be formed on that point by comparing the properties of the plants with the known effects of snake venom. The most obvious of these effects is a paralysis of the motor nerves at the great nerve centres, and as *Acocantherin* strengthens the action of the heart, if the dose is small, this must be supposed to be its action. *Lasiosiphon*, again, is a scorching stimulant, which rouses the powers of life through the stomach, and its use in snake-bite may depend on that. Snake venom, especially the Viperine, also acts as a blood poison, and the Labiate *Leonotis*, and the Acanthaceous *Blepharis* and *Crabbea*, and *Chaetacanthus*, being antiseptics may counteract that effect. The Gentian *Sebaea* would have an action on the blood, and *Cissampelos* is also a blood purifier. The remaining effect of snake-bite is an exceedingly inflamed poisoned wound. The Geraniaceous *Monsonia* has been put forward as a snake-bite remedy, but not on good authority. It is sedative and its only effect would be to keep down inflammation. The envenomed wound ought certainly to be treated with antiseptics as well as with sedatives.

It would be difficult to say how the remaining plants act as antidotes, though it can hardly admit of doubt that they have been of material service.

CHAPTER V.

ANTHRAX OR MILT-ZIEK BLOOD POISONING.

Milt-ziekte, anthrax, or splenic fever, is a fever caused in cattle and sheep by a specific bacillus. In man, as not properly its subject, it occurs in an attenuated form as a blood-poisoning, and the malady is known as malignant pustule, anthrax, malignant carbuncle, milt-ziek blood-poisoning and wool-sorter's disease, and among the Kaffirs as i-dila. The poison enters from eating the flesh of diseased animals, or even using their milk; from getting their blood into a cut or an abrasion of the skin; from handling hides, and, especially at Bradford, from sorting wool taken from sheep which had anthrax. In some cases it has been ascribed to the bite of a gadfly which had been sucking the blood of an animal having this disease; but a supposition so improbable, at least if the person was unconscious of being bitten, merely withdraws attention from the real source of anthrax, which too often is the criminal putting of milt-ziek meat up for sale on the market and in butchers' shops, or making it up into sausages.

Symptoms.—The malady in some cases commences with severe headache, accompanied with pain in the back and limbs, after which, though sometimes before, a pimple appears, if the poison was introduced through eating milt-ziek meat, in any part of the body, and even if it entered externally, the pustule is not necessarily near the point of entrance. This pustule differs from ordinary pimples in being itchy and becoming painful when scratched or squeezed. Subsequently it may be surrounded by a ring of smaller pimples, the heads of which appear watery, and these pimples inflame and swell. The swelling usually goes on extending beyond the part affected, though not invariably so. These symptoms are very irregular in their order of appearing, and one or more of them may be entirely absent. If the malady is treated in time, there may be very little pain felt otherwise, though sometimes headache for one day, In most cases there is a feeling of squeamishness and lassitude, which often is relieved by vomiting. A scab forms over the heads of the pimples, and in favourable cases it rises and drops off, but before it comes off a second has formed.

As angry pimples with a hard lump and suppuration are common enough, which may arise from impurity of blood and are merely boils, people should not imagine that every such pimple is a sign of milt-ziek blood-poisoning, but where swelling goes on extending and those other symptoms are found, it would be advisable to get medical advice at once, as something or other is seriously wrong.

The treatment given here is that of certain native experts, a few among many ignorant empirics, men who are born-doctors, and have also had the transmitted results of long experience. The first step is always to be in time. If the pustule, which under treatment should rise properly, is allowed by delay to go down, a native doctor will not undertake the case, as thinking it useless to do so.

Rationale of the treatment.—The rationale of the treatment is very simple. A decoction, produced by slight simmering, of two bacteria-killing plants controlled by a sedative plant, is given internally in a gradual manner so as to go through the blood and kill poison germs in it, while externally a leaf-paste is made of the same plants to put *around*—not *on*—the pimples, so as to be absorbed and by killing the germs prevent the inflammation from spreading, while that is also reduced by dropping the juice of a sedative plant on the inflamed portion.

Prescription.—One out of many cases successfully treated may be quoted as an example of the native method. The plants were *Blepharis Capensis*, *Cluytia hirsuta*, and *Monsonia ovata*. They are described below.

To administer internally.—Take (Apothecary's Weight):—

Blepharis—of one small plant, including roots	80 grains, or $\frac{1}{8}$ oz.
Cluytia, leaves ...	80 ,, ,, $\frac{1}{6}$ oz.
Monsonia	160 ,, ,, $\frac{1}{3}$ oz.

Simmer or slightly boil in one pint (20 ounces) of water, and administer a tablespoonful six or eight times a day. This must go on till the patient recovers.

For external application.

1 To put *around*, not *on*, the pimples—the same plants but in a different proportion—*Blepharis*, as before $\frac{1}{8}$ oz; but of *Cluytia* and *Monsonia*, only 40 grains or $\frac{1}{12}$ oz of each. The stronger germicide *Blepharis* is made relatively greater in quantity, and the sedative *Monsonia* less, than for internal use, as the stomach cannot bear irritating drugs so well. This application is to be repeated daily.

2 To drop on the pimples—Moisten the leaves of *Monsonia* alone, and squeeze out the juice to make it drop on the pimples. Nothing else ought to touch them. This must go on till the first scab falls off. The patient must be kept quiet and the pustule must not be washed or touched till the first scab comes off, and it is not tied up in any way, but is left exposed to the air. The Kaffir doctors think that the scab must be allowed to drop off without getting the smallest assistance, and believe that death has often been caused by impatience in meddling with it when coming off. They also regard it as fatal to cut or irritate the pustule, while European doctors, on the contrary, frequently cut out the pustule on the idea of preventing the poison from spreading, or they make incisions over the part affected to relieve the tension and the pain. It is matter of notoriety among the Colonists, however, and more so among the Natives, that they have been very unfortunate in their treatment of anthrax, either by allowing it to lapse into a lingering disease, or into a fatal result—and the use of the knife is one mistake. The pustule, like the bubo in the Plague, is not itself the disease, but the effort of nature to throw it out, and it forms a nidus for the bacilli. Were excision employed, or still better, cupping with the Instrument for snake-bite, presently after the poison entered a cut or scratch, that would probably prevent its absorption into the blood, but when in a constitutional disease a pustule is thrown up, the poison must have gone through the blood, and excision is altogether too late. The action taking place from the use of the knife in this case, is paralleled by what happens in inoculation for lung-sickness.

Recently, when inoculation has been gone into generally in this country, the veterinary surgeons used the knife to pare the festered matter from the edges of the wound, and it was found that fresh inflammation was set up and many of the cattle died. They never do so now, though they may wash the wound with hot water. To prevent inflammation from spreading they put a ring of euphorbia milk round the tail above the wound, and the inflammation does not pass that. On the question which treatment of anthrax—the European or the Native,—is the right one, the issue gives the most conclusive verdict. The method followed by European doctors has too often resulted in the death of the patient, whereas the Natives out of confidence in their treatment have the audacity, or rather the madness, to eat milt-ziek meat with a disinfectant, on the presumption that if anything happen they know how to deal with that.

There is a remedy quite on the same lines as this, except that *Withania somnifera, ubu-Vumba*, is substituted for the sedative *Monsonia*; and for internal use an infusion, not a decoction, is made. Perhaps its use is in winter when Monsonia is not to be had. They add a few leaves of Klip dagga.

A third remedy is to use *Cluytia* alone, administering an infusion, and pouring a liquid leaf paste very often on the pimples.

General remarks.—The Kaffir mode of treating anthrax deserves the attention of scientific physicians, even should they have recourse to other drugs superior to those plants. It is based on a dear bought experience, the results of which have been handed down from one generation to another through specialists. Somehow they have groped their way to a treatment which they would have adopted, had they known the germ theory, and they may be said to have had a glimmering of something of the kind, for they proceeded on the idea of combating a poison. They are as jealous of the malignant pustule going down, as medical men are of the rash in scarlet fever doing so, and they leave it and the ring of pimples around it quite bare and exposed to the air, as if they had known that oxygen and sunlight attenuate and even destroy the microbes. They also surround these inflamed parts with antiseptics, which are absorbed and hem in the inflammation in the same manner as is now done in inoculation for lung-sickness with the milk of the euphorbia, and they keep down the inflammation by means of a sedative. Compare this with the mode adopted in a London Hospital of cutting out the pustule four days after it appeared, when it would have been too late to do so at the first moment, for the poison, in a case to be quoted presently, could not have entered by the cheek, and must have already gone through the blood.

The plants they use are proved to be well fitted for arresting anthrax, and as everything in this malady depends on prompt treatment, it would be proper that the plant for milt-ziekte, *Cluytia hirsuta*, should be kept for use in households here, and also exported to England, where in Bradford at least it could be used by wool-sorters on the first symptom of anthrax, and even employed as a prophylactic. It is non-poisonous and safe. The Acanthaceous plants *Blepharis* and *Crabbea* are much stronger, but are probably poisonous, and could not be used with so much confidence.

To put a stop to the inhuman cupidity which leads some persons to kill off animals on the first sign of milt-ziekte and put up the meat for sale, nothing will serve but drastic measures. A section in a public Health Act should make it felony. The same applies to other animal diseases such as lung-sickness, red-water, and quarter-evil, and it will be necessary to have recourse to bacteriology to detect this crime, since discoloration is not the sole criterion of meat being dangerous. The export of milt-ziek skins should also be prohibited unless they can be disinfected.

Cases.—The treatment detailed above was that employed in the case of a Colonist, who had observed a pimple of the ordinary size form on the back of his hand, and feeling it itchy he squeezed it a good deal, which made it feel very painful, and it then began to inflame. Next day he felt lassitude and nausea, followed by the symptoms mentioned before. A native happened to call at his place, and seeing him warned him of milt-ziek poisoning, and advised him to get proper treatment without loss of time; recommending the native doctor, who treated him successfully in the manner described.

A riding-horse which had been employed to carry hides on his back, was poisoned from contact with a milt-ziek skin and died. His owner, a Wesleyan minister, opened the horse to ascertain the cause of death, and got the poison into his blood. He was treated by a European doctor, but the native members of his church, perceiving that he was growing worse, became alarmed for him, and called in a native expert. It was found, however, that the case had gone beyond remedy: their intervention was too late.

A kurveyor in passing through Fort Beaufort lost one of his oxen, from what disease he did not know, but on opening it he found it was milt-ziekte. He did not notice a scratch on his thumb, and was blood-poisoned. He recovered, but it was a three months' case, and he nearly lost his hand. Disagreeable sensations returned for long afterwards in his hand at the same season of the year.

A gentleman in the Customs, and the wife of another employed in the Civil Service, had a pimple, the one in the arm, the other in the lip. The nature of the malady was not perceived until it was too late. There were various conjectures how the poison had got admission, apparently on the supposition that the malignant pustule marks the point of entrance, which is quite a mistake. Probably these valuable lives were lost from milt-ziek meat put on sale.

Four men were working at the London Docks among South African hides, and were blood-poisoned from milt-ziek skins among them. They were taken to St. Bartholomew's Hospital. Two had malignant pustule in the back of the neck and recovered. The other two died from internal ulceration.

The following case affords an illustration of what has already been said on the danger of cutting out the pustule. It was that of a waterside labourer who lived at Bermondsey in London, and the facts are given as stated by his wife at a coroner's inquest. On Friday a small pimple made its appearance on his cheek, but he took no notice of it until the following Monday, when he became very ill and went to the Hospital. At the time the pimple appeared he had been trucking buffalo hides and sheep skins from Gun and Shot Wharf. The hides had been shipped from Penang, and the sheep skins had come from Australia. *An operation was performed and the pustule was cut out.* The deceased appeared to progress favourably. *Secondary inflammation of the neck subsequently set in*, however, *and he gradually sank and died* on the following Friday from blood-poisoning arising from anthrax.

Three native boys near Katberg had eaten milt-ziek meat, which produced a shocking effect on them. They were treated by a native doctor; but whatever his remedies may have been, they seemed to have no effect on one boy who after a time appeared to make no progress, and was enormously swollen. As a last resort the snake-bite cure, a preparation of Red Dagga and ammonia, was tried, after which the swelling fell and the boy began to recover. This is suggestive that in certain cases Dagga—preferably Klip Dagga however—and ammonia may be a valuable auxiliary in the cure of milt-ziek poisoning. Klip Dagga is an element in the second of the remedies given above, and in the cure of blood-poisoning referred to later in this book, and ammonia is an important addition. There are probably instances in which this treatment alone would be sufficient, but the evidence is against relying on it in typical anthrax.

CHAPTER VI.

PLANTS EMPLOYED IN MILT-ZIEK POISONING.

Blepharis Capensis, and *Crabbea cirsioides*—Kaffir, *ubu-Hlungu besigcawu*.
Cluytia hirsuta—Kaffir, *ubu-Hlungu bedila*.
Matricaria nigellaefolia, D C.—Kaffir, *um-Hlonyane womlambo* (river wormwood).
Xanthoxylon Capense, Harv.—*Knobwood, Wild Cardamom*—Dutch, *Paarde praam*—Kaffir, *um-Nungumabele*.
Teucrium Africanum—Dutch, *Padde klauw*—Kaffir, an *ubu-Hlungu benyushu*.

Blepharis Capensis, and *Crabbea cirsioides*—Kaffir, *ubu-Hlungu besiycawu* (Antidote for the tarantula).

These plants belong to closely allied genera of the Acanthaceæ, and are used for the same purposes, and apparently substituted for each other in different parts of the country.

Blepharis C. (eyelash) has a bracteate, 4-divided calyx; corolla with 5 lobes, 3 larger; head of yellow flowers surrounded by numerous bracts, an inch and a half to two inches long, fringed with stiff spinous hairs—hence the name. These bracts when dry and closed together form a head like the dried head of a thistle-like Stobaea, or of some English thistles. The roots are fibrous, and some of them end in tubers. This small plant is found in many places—on the ridge behind Lovedale, at Pirie, on the high ground north of King William's Town, at Main and Clarkebury in Tembuland, and elsewhere.

Crabbea has the calyx 5-parted, with awl-shaped segments; corolla tubular, 5-parted, 3 upper smaller; involucre of stiff, veined, spinous bracts.

In both these, a decoction of the whole plant is used, and a very small quantity is administered, suggesting that more would be dangerous. They are also emloyed as antidotes for the effects of eating diseased meat, other than from *milt-ziekte*, and also in toothache.

Cluytia hirsuta—Kaffir, *ubu-Hlungu bedila.*

This *Cluytia* is an antidote for anthrax, and it also disinfects milt-ziek meat. It is a shrub 3 or 4 feet high, with numerous stems growing up from the same roots. The diœcious flowers are star-like, about a sixth of an inch in diameter, and to be seen properly must be examined with a botanical glass. They have 5 minute white petals, spathulate but hollowed out at the base, with as many 2-3 cleft yellowish glands between them. The segments of the calyx overlap each other, and are green down the centre with a transparent border on each side. The male flower has 5 stamens horizontally attached to a central column. The female flower has three 2-cleft styles. The seed capsules have the form and size of a peppercorn. The leaves are ovate, lanceolate, $1\frac{3}{4}$ inch long by $\frac{3}{8}$ inch wide, and the bark of the newer stems is green.

There is a variety, if it is not a distinct species, growing in the veldt among the grass, 10 inches high or less. The leaves are much smaller than those of the other, 1 inch long by ¾ inch wide. This kind is regarded as superior to the other. The plant belongs to the Order Euphorbiaceae, and apparently has a large amount of quinine, or one of the quinine alkaloids in it, from its giving a green re-action with the chlorine water and ammonia test, and it also has a euphorbia element in the form of an essential oil. Its virtue probably depends on a combination of these. The shrub is found abundantly outside the forests and thickets of the Katberg, and the smaller form is plentiful in the veldt on the slopes facing the south. The natural situation of *C. hirsuta* is in moist, cool, and high localities. I came to know it through the family of B. Knott Esq. of Nottingham, near the Fish River. Some of the children were poisoned with milk from a cow in milt-ziekte, and on an infusion of the leaves being administered to them, they speedily got well. The secret was purchased from a Kaffir servant for the value of ten pounds.

The mode of preparation for administering in milt-ziek poisoning is to make an infusion of the fresh or dried leaves, or to have a tincture in alcohol or brandy in readiness. For external application a liquid leaf-paste is poured on the inflamed parts and that is repeated very often to encourage absorption so as to kill the poison germs. There should always be a supply of the plant in a house. Its value lies in nipping in the bud any poisoning from bad milk or bad meat, and it does not appear to be poisonous itself.

Matricaria nigellaefolia, D C. — Kaffir *um-Hlonyane womlambo* (river-wormwood).

This is a plant abundant in moist ditches and at the edge of pools. It is one of the Compositae, and bears a slight resemblance to the English chamomile. The leaves are twice divided, glaucous; the yellow disc is globose, prominent, and the white ray very short, each petal being only a tenth of an inch long, with a groove down the middle. The plant does not rise above the ground more than three or four inches, but the stems are of some length trailing on the ground and rooting where they touch. It resembles wormwood *(Artemisia Afra)* in its bitter taste and aromatic smell, and slightly in its leaves, and for that reason it has received the name in Kaffir of river-wormwood. Its virtue depends on a bitter principle and essential oil, present chiefly in the flowers.

It is used exactly in the same way as *Cluytia hirsuta* as an antidote for poisoning from *milt-ziekte*. A noted case occured at Bedford of some Kaffirs being poisoned by eating *milt-ziek* meat, who were cured with this plant by an old Fingo doctor.

Xanthoxylon Capense, Harv.—Knobwood, Wild Cardamom—Dutch, *Paarde praam*—Kaffir, *um-Nungumabele.*

The leaves of this shrub or small tree are used for disinfecting *milt ziek* meat, not for curing blood-poisoning. It is common in forests and thickets. The leaf is compound, 4 inches long, with 6 to 8 pairs of opposite leaflets, and a termnial one. The leaflets are ovate, obovate, or lanceolate, with rather distant serratures and a translucent gland in each. The young twigs are covered with short straight spines, and the trunk in larger trees with knobs not unlike a mare's teat, hence the Dutch and Kaffir names. The leaves when rubbed have a strong and peculiar smell. The fruit has a hot pungent taste like pepper, which makes the tip of the tongue tingle.

To disinfect *milt-ziek* meat, they either boil the leaves with the meat, or if they roast the meat, they shred down the leaves to make an infusion with cold water, which they drink along with the meat. This is the most notable of the disinfecting plants, and perhaps the safest, since some of the others have noxious or poisonous properties, at least when used in any quantity. The extent of its power to disinfect is however rendered uncertain from the circumstance that boiling and roasting if thorough would do this work alone.

Teucrium Africanum—Dutch, *Padde klauw*—Kaffir, an *ubu-Hlungu benyushu.*

A notice of this plant is given under the head of SNAKE-BITE PLANTS. It is used to disinfect meat by being boiled along with it.

The following plants are also said to be used for disinfecting milt-ziek meat:—*Withania somnifera*, *ubu-Vumba*; *Solanum nigrum*, Nightshade, *um-Sobo*; and around King William's Town where it is abundant, *Lippia asperifolia*, *in-Zinziniba*; but they have too positive properties as drugs outside of germ-killing, and they are not warranted by any proper Kaffir authority.

CHAPTER VII.

PLANTS USED AS TONICS.

Xysmalobium lapathifolium — Dutch, *Bitter wortel*— Kaffir, *i-Tshongwe.*

Sutherlandia frutescens, R. Br.—Dutch, *Kanker bos.*

Teucrium Africanum—Dutch, *Padde klauw*—Kaffir, an *ubu-Hlungu benyushu.*

Cyperus—Kaffir, *in-Dawa.*

Cluytia hirsuta—Kaffir, *ubu-Hlungu bedila.*

If salts of iron, tincture of calumba, and liquor strychniae are all called Tonics, though their effects are widely different, the first being given to alter the quality of the red blood, the second to give an appetite, and the last to brace the motor nerves, the question arises—What is a tonic? There are no drugs which form a class by themselves under the name of tonics. The definition of a tonic must therefore turn not on some specific character in the drug, but on the intention with which it is administered. It may accordingly be defined to be a medicine, given in in homœopathic quantities over a period, to improve the healthy working of the system. There is always a difficulty in knowing exactly what a tonic can do, but its slow action can be guessed from its effects when administered in quantity for acute disease. The value of this tonic use of a medicine lies in its producing its effects more thoroughly when the person using it can afford to be in no hurry. Those who wish to brace their health with a tonic should never trust to it alone, and relax attention to diet, open air exercise, and the liberal use of water for washing and bathing.

Tonics restore the tone or healthy function, and some of them, if not all, act gently as stimulants. Nothing is more difficult than to say beforehand whether a particular tonic will be beneficial to a person or not; so much depends on constitution, and even on a person's state at the time. The proper way is to make an experiment with the tonic by taking an hour before dinner one dose of 10, or at most 15, minims of a tincture in a little water; or a teaspoonful of a slight decoction, and waiting till the day after the next to note the effects. The unmistakable signs of renewed health are—improved appetite—a feeling of better health and a rise in animal spirits—refreshing sleep—greater bodily warmth especially in the absence of cold hands and feet—insensibility to cold winds and to changes of weather—removal of lassitude—and a craving for work.

Xysmalobium lapathifolium—Dutch, *Bitter wortel*—Kaffir, *i-Tshongwe.*

The genus Xysmalobium bears a considerable resemblance to Gomphocarpus in its general characters, and their medicinal properties are at least related. They agree in the plants being full of a milky juice, and in the follicle or seed-pod being full of a silky cotton. This resemblance is recognised in the popular names given to them of *milk-bush*, *wild cotton*, and in Kaffir *i-tshongwe*. Their roots have a similar and characteristic smell, but differ in form and colour. *Xysmalobium lapathifolium* has the leaves broad, rough, and embracing the stem. Its root is carrot-shaped, straight, long and tapering, and is *very white*, both the inner portion and the bark. The plant grows in moist meadows and sometimes in cultivated fields.

The best way to use the root as a tonic is to grate it down in wine, and after steeping, strain the tincture for use; otherwise, to grate down half a teaspoonful in a little wine.

Sutherlandia frutescens, R. Br.—Dutch, *Kanker bos*.

(See CANCER). A preparation from the leaves of this plant, made in any of the ordinary ways, is employed as a tonic. Its probable function may be presumed from the more pronounced effects of the plant, referred to elsewhere, though its suitability in any case can be found out only by experiment.

Teucrium Africanum—Dutch, *Padde klauw*—Kaffir, an *ubu-Hlungu benyushu*.

This rather notable plant, which is described under SNAKE-BITE, has tonic properties, among its virtues, but it appears to be too peculiar so suit every one. The R. M. and C. C. of Eland's Post speaks highly of it from experience, and he mentions that he recommended its use to a gentleman in shattered health who could neither sleep nor eat, nor walk to his office, but who after using it could do all these with comfort. Any of the modes of preparing the plant will suit, and a few grains will be enough for one dose.

TONICS.

Cyperus—Kaffir, *in-Dawa.*

In-Dawa is a *Cyperus,* found in damp localities, which has running fibrous roots, with knobs, here and there, covered with fibres. The Kaffirs pare these knobs, which are then ½—¾ inch in length, and string them like beads. They are aromatic, pungent like ginger, and bitter, and are used as a tonic, and also in violent colic. The ordinary way is to chew and swallow one or more.

Cluytia hirsuta—Kaffir, *ubu-Hlungu bedila.*

(See MILT-ZIEKTE.) The combination of quinine with a Euphorbiaceous volatile oil in this plant fits it for use of a tonic. Its value would be in cases where there is a torpid condition of stomach and bowels, as the Euphorbia element is stimulating and aperient; but where these are in an irritable state, its use cannot be recommended. A tincture, which might be administered in a little wine, would be most suitable; but two or three leaves reduced to a powder and taken in wine, or the more primitive mode of chewing them and swallowing the juice would serve.

CHAPTER VIII.

PLANTS CONNECTED WITH STOMACH DISORDERS.

Dicoma anomala—Kaffir, *in-Nyongwane*.
Pentanisia variabilis,—Harv.—Kaffir, *i-Rubuxa*.
Sutherlandia frutescens, R. Br.—Dutch, *Kanker bos*.
Alepidea Amatymbica, E. and Z.—Kaffir, *i-Qwili*.
Indigofera (Amecarpus) *patens*.
Indigofera Zeyheri, Spreng.—Dutch, *Leeuw hout*.
Ranunculus Capensis, and *R. pinnatus*.
Mahernia chrysantha, Planch.
Emex spinosa, Campd.—Kaffir, *in-Kunzane*.
Heteromorpha arborescens. Cham. and Schlecht.—Kaffir, *um-Bangandlela*.

Dicoma anomala—Kaffir *in-Nyongwane*.

This is one of the Compositæ. The leaves are linear, pointed, rough but without hairs above, woolly beneath, finely serrate, margin slightly revolute. The involucre is composed of numerous series of awlshaped pointed leaflets, the inner gradually longer. The flower is purple, and the seed-down white, consisting of slender bristles seen under a botanical glass to be bordered with fine hairs. The rootstock is woody. The plant is plentiful at Main in Tembuland.

The leaves of *in-nyongwane* are intensely bitter. The

plant is used for various purposes. For colic a little of the powdered root is administered in cold water. It is also employed for a very singular purpose. If a Kaffir goes to a strange place, he chews a little of the root, so that if he receive any poisoned food he may immediately vomit it. Probably its best use has yet to be ascertained.

Pentanisia variabilis, Harv.—Kaffir, *i-Rubuxa*, and in Tembuland, *ili-Dliso*—Fingo, *isi-Cimamlilo*.

This plant is very common on the Katberg, especially on some of the spurs, and is also found on Chumie Peak. Although it grows among the grass and is not a large plant, it is very conspicuous from its head of small flowers which are dark purple or dark blue on the corolla tube, and outside of the limb except at the margin, and lilac, or light blue in the inside, a similar combination of colours to that in agapanthus, and having the same sombre look. The flowers form an umbel-like spike on a four-sided or compressed stalk. The corolla is salver-shaped with a tube an inch long, and a limb of five lobes. The root is large, 3—4 inches long and an inch or more in diameter, but occasionally it is very much longer. *I-Rubuxa* is the proper name in Kaffir. *Ili-Dliso* is neither common nor confined to this plant. It is called *isi-Cimamlilo* (ukucima to extinguish, umlilo fire), because it is one of the plants used according to a superstition to remove the effects of lightning-stroke.

The root, which is the part used, appears to have properties related to those of ipecacuanha. In cases of swelling of the stomach, the root is bruised and boiled, and the decoction is mixed with sour milk and drunk. The decoction is also drunk for retarded after-birth, and for this is also given to animals.

Sutherlandia frutescens, R. Br.—Dutch, *Kanker bos*.

(See CANCER.) A case given here in the manner and language of the persons concerned, should be suggestive of an important use to which Sutherlandia may be turned. It was of an erf-holder, who neither cultivated, nor did any other sort of work, and was regarded as a lazy person. His wife, however, said her husband was not well, and was unable to work. He had a feeling of extreme weakness and sinking at the stomach, the effect of a malady peculiarly defiant of medical treatment. He left the locality for a time along with his family and when he returned, his wife said of her husband that he was another man now, and they would not know him again. The remedy he used was homely enough. A pinch of the leaves of Sutherlandia was put into a cup and boiling water was poured on them. He took a little of this infusion twice or thrice a day, and became quite strong and was now doing heavy work. If any symptom of the former weakness returned, a little of the same removed it. The action of Sutherlandia on the system in this instance is probably similar to that in the case mentioned under Dysentery, though the symptoms of the disorder are different.

Alepidea Amatymbica, E. and Z.—Kaffir, *i-Qwili.*—Dutch, *Kalmoes.*

Alepidea ciliaris. L. Roche—Dutch, *Berg Kalmoes.*

A. Amatymbica is an Umbellifer with the general umbels irregular though the partial umbels are regular.

The stem is 2—4 feet high, the root-leaves are 6—15 inches long, 1½—3 inches wide, toothed, with a bristle ⅛ inch long at the point of each tooth; the stem leaves grow smaller upwards. The root-stock is large, covered with a brown bark; is white when freshly cut, but the cut surface presently turns reddish brown. It is resinous and very bitter, and has a strong peculiar smell.

A. ciliaris is a small species found on mountains. It is usually from 12 to 20 inches high, but is sometimes of a larger growth if it chance to be in a moist spot with deep soil. The flowers are white; the root-leaves are on stalks, those on the stem are clasping, and all are fringed with stiff hairs, as the name of the species implies. This species is employed as a medicine for cattle.

There are varieties of the two species just named, which have undergone considerable modification from situation, but are unworthy of being ranked as distinct species. At the same time there are one or two which have neither been described nor named, and which are undoubtedly different species. One is reported as growing in Griqualand East, found in shady places on hill sides. The leaf is dark green on the upper side and silvery white below.

No other species answers to these characters, and it is believed to be more reliable than those mentioned. The dose is a tea-spoonful of the powdered root.

A small dose of *i-qwili* is administered for pain in the stomach or abdomen. A large dose is purgative. Small doses of the root have tonic properties. For use, a portion of the root may be powdered and given in cold water; or a tincture may be made. Great care must be taken in regard to quantity, as the Umbellifers are frequently dangerous. As an example of its use, an intelligent European farmer had suffered from a severe form of measles, and during recovery was suddenly seized with colic-like abdominal pain, and on domestic remedies failing, resorted to the root of *i-qwili*, got from a Kaffir source. A small tea-spoonful of the root finely powdered and administered, removed all pain in half an hour.

A case of colic cured by *i-qwili* may be placed here as originating in eating a quantity of most indigestible food, though it took the form of a dysenteric diarrhœa. It was that of a young farmer with whom the attack became so violent as to cause protrusion of the bowel. He was cured with *kalmoes*, but after rallying the first time he revolted against the regimen of a milk diet, and brought on a second attack which nearly cost him his life.

Indigofera (Amecarpus) patens, E. and Z.

A small shrublet plentiful on the ridge behind Lovedale, also near the Philipton river, and elsewhere; found in dry stony ground. The leaves are sessile, trifoliolate, leaflets 2—4 lines long, 1—2 wide, flowers small, bright scarlet, very fugitive. The root which goes straight down is large for the size of the plant, woody, with a taste at first like the roots of many other leguminous plants, but presently showing a pronounced bitter.

A decoction of the roots is employed when people have a loathing for food, or are troubled with indigestion. If bile has gone through the body, the Kaffir doctors say that the decoction produces a rash in a very short time. It is an appetite producing plant and is diuretic. The plant is dangerous, and if used at all, it should be in the smallest quantity.

Indigofera Zeyheri, Spreng.—Dutch, *Leeuw hout.*

Unlike the former, which is found in a dry climate, this plant is found in a climate which is humid either from elevation, or from proximity to the sea. It is plentiful on the south side of the Katberg, and at Main in Tembuland. The leaves are 3—5 jugate, leaflets rough with appressed bristles pointing forward, mucronate. The root is large for the plant, rather spongy. The flowers are purple. The root is chewed to remove flatulence.

This plant is mentioned here to guard against its use even in so trifling a quantity. A Kaffir empiric administered a pannikin of a decoction made from the root to a woman in sickness, with a fatal result, for which deservedly he was criminally punished. In connection with his trial, experiments were made on animals with a decoction. They exhibited signs of stupor and paralysis. The property which produces this appears to run through the Indigoferas. The cakes of blue, formerly used with wash clothes, were of indigo, not of prussian blue, and they were employed to deaden the pain from the stings of bees and wasps.

Ranunculus Capensis, and *R. pinnatus*.

A plant will sometimes effect a cure, when the medicines of the regular course fail. A young patient was affected with vomiting and such extreme irritability of stomach that it retained nothing he swallowed, not even a little water. This state of matters lasted for three days. The leaves of the Ranunculus were slightly boiled, and the decoction was allowed to cool and sweetened. Two table-spoonfuls were administered, and repeated after two hours. This entirely removed the disorder. The juice of the Ranunculus is acrid, and most likely this is the efficacious property in such a case; but caution must be used as to the quantity of leaves employed, in case of serious mischief being done by a strong decoction. Probably several of the species of Ranunculus would do.

It is well worthy of trial whether a tincture of Ranunculus leaves would allay the irritability of stomach which causes sea-sickness. Probably it would.

Mahernia chrysantha, Planch.

Is a plant with stalked oblong leaves, sub-cordate at the base, becoming smooth above, but woolly beneath. The flower is yellow. It is used for colic by the Basutos.

Emex spinosa Campd.—Kaffir, *in-Kunzane*.

This plant grows in gardens and cultivated fields, and is so well known, that the slightest description will be sufficient for identifying it. Its leaves remind one of the dock, it has a red fleshy root, and produces a globular fruit, as large as a pea, furnished on opposite sides with three formidable spines, very awkward to tread on with the naked foot.

The leaves are boiled and used as a cabbage in dyspepsia, and in biliousness, and also for creating an appetite. They are mildly purgative, and diuretic.

Heteromorpha arborescens, Cham. and Schlecht.—Kaffir, *um-Bangandlela*.

For a notice of the plant, see under SCROFULA.

A tincture, or an infusion of the inner bark and of the bark of the roots is used for colic.

CHAPTER IX.

PLANTS USED IN HEALING WOUNDS AND SORES.

Aloe saponaria, or *latifolia*, Haw.—*White-spotted Aloe*—Kaffir, *in-Gcelwane*.
Pelargonium alchemilloides, Willd—[with *Malva parviflora*, Linn.—Kaffir, *u-Nomolwana*.]
Hibiscus aelthiopicus, Linn.
Lasiosiphon Meisneri—Kaffir, *isi-Dikili*.
The common Arum.
Amygdalis Persica—The Peach.
Xysmalobium lapathifolium—Kaffir, *i-Tshongwe*.
Pelargonium reniforme, Curt.—Kaffir, *i-Yeza lezikali*.
Helichrysum pedunculare, D C.—Kaffir, *isi-Cwe*.
Venidium arctotoides, Less.—Kaffir, *ubu-Shwa*.
Urtica—The Nettle—Kaffir, *i-Rau*
Senecio latifolius—Kaffir, *i-Dwara*.
Senecio concolor, D C.—Kaffir, *um-Dambiso*.
Withania somnifera—Kaffir, *ubu-Vumba*.
Melianthus comosus—Dutch, *Kruidje roer mij niet*.

The healing of wounds is nature's work, but plants in different ways are an aid. Some have merely a soothing, healing virtue. Others draw out inflammation, and others again have a pungency which quickens wounds that have gone into a dead state. Then there are those which like carbolic acid kill germs, and there are also styptics, and those that kill maggots bred in sores.

Aloe saponaria, or *latifolia*, Haw.—*White spotted Aloe*—
    Kaffir *in-Gcelwane*.

The common medicinal Aloe with its tall spike of red flowers is well known in the Eastern Province. The white-spotted Aloe has a leaf of the same size and thickness, with similar prickles at the edges, but it is a low plant comparatively, and the leaves are covered with white markings. There are two varieties, or possibly species, answering to this description, which differ in the form of the flowers and flower-stalk, as well as in the white markings on the leaves; and the amber coloured juice, which oozes out at the base of the leaves, turns after exposure to the air to a bright purple in the one, and to a dull purple in the other. The two have the same healing properties. This is perhaps the best of all the plants which have a virtue in healing an inflamed wound. It acts at once and begins by changing the colour of the wound. The value of the plant is also great in severe burns. It requires no preparation. The leaf is cut open and applied to a wound. In fresh cuts it is equally serviceable. As pungency is an element in the cure of wounds, the yellow aloetic juice found only at the base of the leaf should be employed as well as the transparent juice. With regard to burns, it appears to be hardly known, that the most effective way to keep down inflammation is to hold the burnt part long under water rather colder than the temperature of the blood. It may take some trouble to keep the water at the proper temperature, for warm water and decidedly cold water both increase the inflammation. Still it might be the means of saving life in some cases. The application of rags moistened with cold water will not serve the same purpose.

This aloe is employed for ring-worm, and the yellow juice is preferable in this use also.

Pelargonium alchemilloides, Willd.—Kaffir, an *in-Kubele*
—[with *Malva parviflora*, Linn.—Kaffir, *u-Nomolwana*.]

This Pelargonium is altogether herbaceous, with kidney-shaped, 5—7 lobed leaves on long leaf-stalks. The leaves are pubescent, beautifully soft and velvety, with a dark horse-shoe in the middle of the leaf. Another species is found growing along side of it in some localities, also herbaceous and marked with the horse-shoe, but the leaf is hard and the lobes are different. Many specimens of both species are found without the dark marking on the leaf, and in other common species of Pelargonium the same leaf-marking is found, but they have woody stems. *In-Kubele* is a generic term for healing plants, including some of the Pelargoniums.

Malva, the Mallow, is a common weed, with kidney-shaped 5—7 lobed crenate leaves, found near hedges, and varying extremely in size from being a plant two or three inches high to be as many feet. The flowers are of a pale rose-colour.

These two plants should be used in combination. When any part is swollen and inflamed, or when a wound festers, a paste of mallow leaves—either warmed or not—is applied, which quickly draws out the inflammation, and brings the abscess to a point. A wound is also washed with a decoction of mallow leaves, made in an earthenware vessel, not in a metal pot.

After a wound is properly drawn by the mallow leaf-paste, a paste of the leaves *P. alchemilloides* will heal it quickly.

The case of a youth at an Educational Institution will show the use of this Pelargonium. He had a bad sore in the upper part of his foot caused by the poisonous dye from a sock getting into an abrasion of the skin, which ended in a cavity being made there and one in the hollow of his foot as well. The visiting doctor on seeing it, said his foot would require to be taken off. As the young student did not relish that, he went home, and after some poulticing the juice from the moistened leaves of this plant was repeatedly squeezed into the wounds. That went on for some time, and in a month he returned to his studies, not without his foot, but with it perfectly cured.

This Pelargonium is found in abundance on the right bank of the Chumie opposite Lovedale, and in the Swelamanzi (Water-less) valley near the same spot; also at Balfour in Kat River, and is widely distributed.

Hibiscus aethiopicus, Linn.

A Hibiscus is so readily recognized by anyone who knows a single species, that a generic description is not necessary, and only the distinguishing marks of the species H. aethopicus are given here. This is a low lying plant, found on ridges among the grass, 6 or 8 inches long, with elliptical leaves irregular in shape, sometimes entire, otherwise notched, having 3 or 5 ribs, and covered especially at the margin and on the ribs with bristles radiating star-like from the same point. The style is elongated beyond the staminal tube enclosing it, is 5-cleft, each division ending in a globular purple brush. The flowers are axillary, bright yellow with a purple centre, and not opening fully so as to lie flat. A yellow tinge runs through the whole plant. In this Section of the genus Hibiscus, the involucel beneath the lobes of the calyx consists of 10—12 awl-shaped leaflets.

One would hardly imagine a common weed like this to be of any service in serious wounds, yet it appears to be otherwise from a case where the sole of a person's foot was pierced by treading on a piece of fencing wire. which produced a bad wound with great swelling and with the inflammation coming out above. The wound was washed with hot water and carbolic soap, and another healing plant was tried, without effect. On a liquid leaf-paste of this Hibiscus being applied, the excessive swelling went down, and next day this person could walk about.

The result will appear less wonderful, when it is known that the Hibiscus belongs to the Malvaceae, and may be presumed to have a virtue in drawing inflammation out of a wound like the common Mallow. No Hottentot could possibly have divined that this plant belongs to the Mallow Family, a proof that their medicinal knowledge is largely experimental. Other species of the same genus, such as *H. pusillus* and *H. Trionum* probably have a similar property, and it may in some degree run through the whole genus.

Lasiosiphon Meisneri—Kaffir, *isi-Dikili*.

(See SNAKE-BITE.) *Isi-Dikili* has a considerable range in its uses. Its virtue depends on an extremely pungent quality running through the plant, though chiefly in the root, and on another principle less perceptible on account of the strength of the former. It is a plant of great value in wounds and sores of every kind, and in eruptions from impurity of blood.

For external application it is of special use in old sores, where its efficacy is due to the quickening effects of its pungency; but it may be employed in wounds of any sort. To prepare a salve for the purpose, an intimate blend may be made of the root reduced to an impalpable powder and lard, or vaseline. It would also serve, to make a strong tincture of the root and unite this with olive oil, or an animal oil. Either preparation should be well rubbed in.

A paste of the leaves will also heal wounds and sores.

Its internal use is perhaps more important. It has singular power as a remedy for foul eruptions of various kinds, even for some sort of leprosy causing the loss of toes, for abnormal growths and gatherings, and for sores which obstinately resist healing. All these arise from blood impurities, and its action here is that of a blood purifier. A preparation may be made from the root, after finely dividing it, by tincture, by slight decoction, or by infusion either hot or cold. The strength and the quantity to use are somewhat indeterminate, for its pungency being at least as great as that of cayenne pepper, especially in the time it lasts, what would suit one person would do mischief to another with a more sensitive and delicate mucous membrane. It is always better to begin low, and one can judge how it will affect the stomach which does not feel, by the degree in which it scorches the tonsils and the throat. The root should always be used tolerably fresh, as it loses its virtue by long keeping.

The other species of Lasiosiphon, L. linifolius, and L. anthylloides have similar properties, but are of less value.

A case may be given to show the action of *isi-dikili*. The following is of an English farmer resident in the district of Komgha. He had hurt his leg, and the effect of the injury remained for three or four years, turning during the last year and a half to a sore which eventually necessitated an operation. The sore healed for some months and then broke out again, occasioned obviously by impurity of blood. He was induced, though with reluctance, to try a preparation of *isi-dikili* used internally, and the effect being favourable both on the sore and on his health, he persevered for a length of time, with the result that the sore disappeared and his general health was much improved. *Isi-dikili* acted in this instance only as a blood-purifier, and the case being chronic the remedy required time to take effect. This principle will apply to all blood-purifying, and the rule to be followed should be to effect it by a slow action with small doses over an extended period.

The common Arum, or The Egyptian lily (Richardia Africana, or Calla Aethiopica.)

This plant though not native is now found in moist places everywhere. It has a special value in sores which require drawing, as will appear from an instance in point. In dissecting for what proved to be a case of sponsziekte (quarter-evil), a post-contractor got some of the black poisonous matter found internally, into a chink beneath his finger nail. His arm became extremely swollen, and he began to show symptoms of coma. To arrest that, incisions were made in his arm into which Croft's Tincture was put, and it was also given internally. He was forcibly kept awake the following night, and next day he felt relieved, but ulceration went on in his arm, and it was carried in a sling for two months. A Dutch farmer recommended him to throw away the linseed poultices, and wrap scorched Arum leaves round his arm, changing them every hour. Heat makes the leaves soft and flaccid. This application had a magical effect in healing the ulcers. The arum has a great power in drawing. Its juice is poisonous, and a small piece of the bulbous root swallowed will produce swelling in the tongue and constriction in the muscles of the throat, and other more dangerous effects.

While the ulcers consequent on sponsziek poisoning were healed by the arum, it would be of no use to arrest the the poisoning at the outset, nor can Croft's Tincture, though serviceable, be relied on for that. The same treatment as in milt-ziek blood-poisoning would probably be suitable. This will be referred to farther on under Blood-poisoning.

Amygdalis Persica—The Peach.

The leaves of the Peach have some very important uses, due to the presence of prussic acid the most powerful sedative known. There was a little boy, on whose chest a fly blister had inadvertently been left to remain too long. On its removal, his breast became enormously swollen, with an ugly sore under his throat, and as he could not lie, he sat moaning with his head bent down. A decoction of peach leaves was applied. In half-an-hour the child ceased to moan, in an hour the swelling was gone, and next day his breast was almost well. This indicates that peach leaves have an unusual power of reducing inflamed wounds.

A decoction of peach leaves has also a remarkable virtue in reducing the inflammation and clearing out the matter in an ugly sore, at the same time removing the offensive smell. Whether it also can kill the poison germs in gangrenous sores, remains to be seen. It would be a discovery of importance, were that found to be the case.

In this country a decoction of peach leaves is used for destroying maggots in sores, and they are got rid of without injury to the parts.

While prussic acid is most probably the active agent in all these cases, it does not follow that the acid in a very dilute form would produce the same effects. Nature blends her curative agents with their necessary complements in so delicate a manner that art cannot imitate it.

Xysmalobium lapathifolium—Kaffir, *i-Tshongwe*.

A description of this plant is given under TONICS. In hot climates maggots are apt to breed in festering wounds, and it is troublesome to destroy them without injuring the parts. The milk of *X. lapathifolium* is efficacious, and this is the best species, though the other species and those of *Gomphocarpus* will do. *I-Tshongwe* is a generic term for all these.

Pelargonium reniforme, Curt.—Kaffir, *i-Yeza lezikali.*

The leaves of this Pelargonium are of a blueish green, kidney-shaped, lobed or crenate, velvety above, cottony and with very prominent nerves beneath, and they are on long stalks. There are two varieties, which are used by the Kaffirs, one with rose purple flowers with a dark purple spot at the base of the two upper petals; the other with flowers of a dark port-wine colour.

The leaves when boiled yield a mucilage which is made use of to keep the air out of a wound, and also to prevent the eggs from being deposited, which produce maggots.

Helichrysum pedunculare, D C.—Kaffir, *isi-Cwe.*

The Kaffir *abakweta,* youths undergoing circumcision, use the leaves of *isi-cwe.* This plant is believed to have the power to keep down dangerous inflammations. The woolly underside of the leaf is put next a wound. The flower-stalk is tall, with a cyme of many heads of yellow flowers. The root-leaves are large, dark-green and glossy above, woolly and white beneath. It is found in the pastures.

Venidium arctotoides, Less.—Kaffir, *ubu-Shwa*—Dutch, *Goud bloem (Gold flower.)*

This is one of the Compositae. The heads are yellow with the florets of the disk 5-toothed, perfect; those of the ray, strap-shaped, female. The leaves are stalked, lyrate, pinnatifid, more or less woolly and white beneath. It is plentiful almost everywhere.

The leaves have the power of healing some kinds of

wounds with great rapidity. They have a pungent, burning quality, producing a smart sensation at first, and are best fitted for old sores. The mode of using the plant, followed by the Kaffirs, is to freshen the sore by scratching, and then squeeze out the juice upon it, or apply a leaf-paste. A variety of larger growth found in moist places is called river *ubu-shwa*, and is milder.

Urtica—The Nettle—Kaffir, an *i-Rau*.

The plant referred to here is not the introduced European nettle, which may however have similar properties, but the small native nettle with tender leaves, one or two species of which are found in the Eastern Districts. A leaf-paste of this nettle is of great value for its healing properties, and amongst other uses it is employed in cases where the eyelids are red all over. So much is the plant esteemed, that some Dutch colonists have handed down a knowledge of its value in healing as a family tradition.

Plantago—The Plantain.

As in England, the leaves of the plantain—Cape species—are applied in this country to wounds, especially to sores in the legs.

Senecio latifolius, var. *barbellatus*—Kaffir, *i-Dwara*.

A very common Composite plant, the yellow flowers in a panicle, lower leaves oblong, acute, clasping at the base, upper leaves narrow and entire at the edge. A paste of the leaves is employed for burns, and also for wounds.

WOUNDS AND SORES.

Senecio concolor, D C.—Kaffir, *um-Dambiso*

This plant is covered with soft jointed hairs, has the lower leaves toothed, oblong; the upper leaves narrower; the root leaves are lyrate, and lobed. The flowers are few, with the disk and the ray purple.

The leaves are made into a paste and used for cuts and wounds to keep down inflammation and swelling.

Withania somnifera—Kaffir, *ubu-Vumba*—Fingo, *u-Vimba*

(SEE ANIMAL MEDICINES.) An ointment of real efficacy in healing wounds and sores is prepared by some of the Colonists from this plant by boiling the leaves in lard.

Melianthus comosus—Dutch, *Kruidje roer mij niet.*

A poultice or paste for cleansing bad sores, and for swollen bruises is made from the leaves. It reduces the swelling very quickly.

CHAPTER X.

PLANTS USED IN BLOOD-PURIFYING.

Bulbine aloöides, and *Bulbine latifolia*—Dutch, *Rooi wortel* —Kaffir, an *in-Gcelwane*.

A foreign element in the blood is called a blood-impurity. It may be an acid, or bile, or a poison-germ, or something else, things which having nothing in common require a totally different treatment; and a false impression is given when a blood purifier is put forward and alleged to remove all impurities of the blood, when each may necessitate a different remedy.

These plants have hardly a stem. The leaves are broad, embracing, without prickles. The flower stalk is 12—20 inches high, with a raceme of bright yellow flowers, perianth 6-parted, stamens bearded at the top. The tuber is orange-yellow, the older parts redder. It yields a beautiful carmine tincture.

These characters apply to more species than one, but so far as the broad leafed section of this genus has been described by the earlier botanists, the species have been mixed up and confused both in names and in description. One of the two referred to here is very like an aloe, with leaves broad at the base, very fleshy and watery, and tapering to a point. The leaves of the other are elongate elliptical, firmer, and of a lighter green. The tubers according to the age of the plant vary in size from that of a walnut to be as large as yams. They are very bitter, and these species have similar properties.

Rooi wortel is placed under the head of blood-purifying, though given here for rheumatism, specially that following rheumatic fever, since its efficacy in this malady, as well as in weakness of heart and of the involuntary muscles, is due in part at least to its action as a blood purifier.

Ordinary rheumatism is occasioned by a want of vigour in the circulation of the blood, which appears from its being brought on at once, or aggravated, by the depressing effect of damp weather. The rheumatism consequent on rheumatic fever, left after the fever is gone, though there is a concomitant weakness in the circulation, is attributed to the presence of lactic acid in the blood, and it is at this point that Bulbine comes in as a blood purifier to remove the impurity. Its power to do so has been tested in numerous cases, both of Europeans and of Natives, with the result that the rheumatism is removed, and the impaired vigour of the circulation is restored. The latter can result only from its invigorating the heart, and that applies also to the peristaltic action. How the drug acts to effect this is matter of opinion. It may do so by preventing, or even removing, a deposit which weakens the involuntary muscles; but the fact remains, whatever view may be taken of the cause.

Much circumspection is required in the use of Bulbine. Like *salicin* it produces a depression, which will not therefore disprove its efficacy in cases of weak heart, but which necessitates great caution as to quantity. Used for any purpose, too large a dose may produce a diarrhœa, while a small dose checks that and tends to produce constipation. The drug may also occasion acidity and flatulence. Any one of these things, unless corrected, may defeat the main object. The proper dose is 10 minims of a tincture in which the dried tuber is to the solvent as 1 to 8 (a drachm to a fluid oz.), taken in a little water, and the safe way is to begin with one dose half an hour before dinner, and taking none the next day, wait till the following morning to observe the effects. If the resulting action has been favourable, despite of a depression on the day before, a person can then take a dose daily, and go on to twice a day, if that is found desirable.

The use of Bulbine as a blood purifier is not restricted to the removal of lactic acid, but is general, and it will remove the purplish colour from the blood and restore the bright red colour. It cannot be said at present how far it will go as a remedy for weak heart. If it prove to be so, it will be an important drug, and all the more that its effect, unlike that of strychnine or strophanthin, would be not merely to strengthen the action of the heart, but to remove the cause of weakness. Trial should be made of this drug to remove the taint or dregs left by the cholera and influenza poisons.

There are other blood-purifiers specific rather than general, and they are ranked under those heads which express their special function. *Heteromorpha, um-Bangandlela*, is placed under Scrofula; *Lasiosiphon, isi-Dikili*, under Sores and eruptions; *Cissampelos, Davidjes*, under Syphilitic poisoning; and *Sutherlandia, Kanker bos*, under Cancer.

CHAPTER XI.

PLANTS USED FOR SCROFULA.

It has been remarked that the Kaffirs seldom apply to European doctors for scrofula, though that malady is common among them, which suggests that they have found effective remedies of their own. Some of the remedies are given below.

Heteromorpha arborescens, Cham. and Schlecht.—Kaffir, *um-Bangandlela.*

Zizyphus mucronata, Willd.—*The Wait-a-bit thorn-tree—um-Pafa.*

Bulbine asphodeloides, Schult.—Dutch, *Wilde Capive* (Copaiba)—Fingo, an *i-Yeza lehashe.*

{ *Silene Burchellii*, Ott.—Kaffir, an *i-Yeza lehashe.*
{ *Rubia petiolaris*, D C.—Dutch, *Rooi houtje.*

{ *Pentanisia variabilis*, Harv.—Kaffir, *i-Rubuxa.*
{ *Erythrina Humei*, E. Mey.—*Small Kaffir-tree*—Kaffir, *um-Sintsana.*
{ *Eriosema salignum*, E. Mey.—Kaffir, *um-Fisi.*
{ *Rhyncosia gibba*, E. Mey.—Kaffir, *i-Yeza lomoya olubomvu.*

Solanum Capense—Kaffir, *um-Tumana.*

Thunbergia Capensis, Thun.—Kaffir, an *i-Yeza lehashe.*

Heteromorpha arborescens, Cham. and Schlecht.—Kaffir *um-Bangandlela.*

This *umbellifer* is a small tree, a rare thing in this Order. It is plentiful on the Katberg, and in the valleys of the Chumie and the Gaga, near the rivers. The flower is yellowish, the fruit three winged. The leaves vary in different specimens and are tri-foliolate, three lobed or parted, ovate and pointed. The bark is almost unique. The outer bark is of a drab colour, shining, and is divided at distances of one or more inches by rough rings, found to a slight extent next below this bark, but not in the wood. The outer bark is leathery and is easily separated. The middle bark is of a beautiful green, and inner the bark is very white.

This is a rather important plant in Kaffir use. The parts employed are the inner bark and the bark of the roots. For scrofula, they are slightly boiled, the decoction is allowed to cool, and is used internally three times a day. It is said, that if it is used for a week, the scrofula passes off in the secretions, and the running ceases; while swellings on the chest break and come out.

Zizyphus mucronata, Willd.—*The Wait-a-bit thorn-tree*—Kaffir, *um-Pafa*.

The Wait-a-bit thorn, which grows to the size of a large tree, with its recurved prickles and red fruit the size of a wild cherry, is so well known in Kaffraria, Kat River, and elsewhere in the Eastern districts as to need no description.

The root is glutinous and a decoction of it is used internally for all scrofulous diseases, and for swollen glands of the neck. A paste of the leaves is also applied to glandular swellings.

Bulbine asphodeloides, Schult.—Dutch, *Wilde Capive (Copaiba)*—Fingo, one of several plants called *i-Yeza lehashe*—Kaffir, *in-Telezi.*

The Bulbines all have a perianth with six segments, and the filaments of the stamens very hairy at the top giving the bright yellow flowers a peculiar and striking appearance. The head of flowers in this species forms a bunch on a stalk a foot high. The dark green leaves, 10 inches long, $\frac{1}{5}$ inch broad, and $\frac{1}{8}$ inch thick, are clustered round the flower-stalk with the flat side towards it, and resemble a bunch of shalots. The bulbous rootstock has a large bundle of roots attached to it. Its juice and that of the leaves will readily give anything a yellow stain. The natural situation of the plant is in high and moist localities. It is easily distinguished from B. longiscapa, which has a flower-stalk with the flowers sparsely distributed over six or eight inches at the top, and lighter coloured leaves with a bloom on them, much resembling those of an onion.

A decoction or other preparation made from the fleshy bulbous portion, the rootstock, and the roots, is employed in scrofula. It belongs to a blood-purifying family, and it appears to have a special adaptation for removing the scrofula impurity. As in all blood-purifying drugs the quantity used ought to be small, and to extend over a considerable period.

Silene Burchellii, Ott.—Kaffir, an *i-Yeza lehashe.*
Rubia petioloris, D C.—Dutch *Rooi houtje.*

This *Silene,* a *Catchfly,* has flesh-coloured petals, the

calyx ¾ inch long, with green striæ, the upper leaves nearly linear, roots perennial.

Rubia petiolaris, See DYSENTERY.

These plants are sometimes called *i-Yeza lehashe*, but that is a general term, not distinctive. When the *Silene* is used alone, a hot infusion is made from the bruised roots, and this is taken internally once a day.

If the *Rubia* is added, the roots of both are bruised in cold water, and the infusion taken once a day.

Pentanisia variabilis, Harv.—Kaffir, *i-Rubuxa*, and in Tembuland *ili-Dliso*—Fingo, *isi-Cimamlilo*
Erythrina Humei, E. Mey.—*Small Kaffir-tree*—Kaffir, *um-Sintsana*.
Eriosema salignum, E. Mey.—Kaffir, *um-Fisi*.
Rhyncosia gibba, E. Mey.—Kaffir, *i-Yeza lomoya olubomvu*.

For *i-Rubuxa*, See STOMACH.

The small Kaffir-tree is so well known as to need no description. *E. Humei* may be distinguished from the larger and coarser shrub *E. Zeyheri* by its glossy smaller leaves 2—3 inches long, its leaf-stalks and sometimes the nerves of the leaves being prickly, and by its crimson-scarlet flowers.

For *um-Fisi*, See KIDNEYS.

Rhyncosia gibba is a leguminous plant with trailing pubescent stems, leaflets round or rhomboid, the upper petal of the flowers streaked with brown, the pod falcate. These four plants are used together for scrofula. The roots of the first two, *i-rubuxa* and *um-sintsana* are bruised and boiled for a fomentation, and a little of the decoction is also drunk. The fomentation opens the pores, and the leaves of the second two—*um-fisi* and *iyeza lomoya olubomvu*—reduced to a powder are rubbed on the scrofulous swellings.

Solanum Capense—Kaffir, *um-Tumana*. (See DISTEMPER.)

The leaves are used for scrofula. They are bruised and infused in hot water, and the infusion is used for bathing the parts affected; after which a paste of the fresh leaves is applied as a poultice.

Thunbergia Capensis, Thun.—Kaffir, an *i-Yeza lehashe*.

In this plant the corolla is orange yellow with a swollen throat and a 5-lobed limb. The calyx is concealed under two large bracts. The leaves are oval, with prominent ribs on the back, diverging from the base of the leaf, but also branched; very rough and hairy on both sides, as are also the leaf and flower stalk. It is found in Tembuland.

The leaves mixed with those of *i-tyolo* (clematis) and *um-pafa* (wait-a-bit thorn) are bruised and applied to scrofulous swellings.

CHAPTER XII.

TYPHOID FEVER—RHEUMATIC FEVER—INFLUENZA.

TYPHOID FEVER.

Typhoid or enteric fever is prevalent in South Africa, and is sometimes epidemic among the natives in certain localities especially in years of drought, a result traceable to bad water. The plant resources available in typhoid are few, as the germ-killers, so efficacious in blood-poisoning, are too acrid and irritant for use in a malady with an internal eruption. The Hottentots accordingly have recourse to a distant relative of Chamomile as a fever medicine.

Matricaria globifera, Fenzl.—Dutch, *Meste kruid*.

The flower heads of this Composite are yellow, as the disk in this class usually is, globular, and destitute of rays. As in chamomile, they form the more important part of the plant. The leaves are extremely subdivided, and narrow linear. The whole plant is very bitter and has a heavy smell due to its being charged with an essential oil, on which along with a bitter principle its virtue depends. A preparation from it can certainly be made very strong, which is some comfort to those who are excluded from anything better. It grows near kraals and among the sweet grass beside cattle lairs—hence its Dutch name. The usual preparation is a hot infusion of the fresh flowers and leaves, or of each separately, and they are kept also in the dried state, as the plant dies away and disappears before midsummer.

When doctors give directions what people in sickness should do, when they order this and interdict the other thing, they rarely state the reason why; and that applies to typhoid fever more than to most things. Their alleged motive is to avoid creating alarm; the real reason probably is their wish to keep the key of knowledge to themselves. In typhoid fever they interdict all solids, especially potatoes, bread, and farinaceous food, and give directions that the patient get nothing but beef-tea and milk; but they give no reason why. The reason why is this. Enteric fever has its eruption in a portion of the small bowel, where there is intense inflammation, and the membrane sometimes becomes thin. Anything solid passing this point may aggravate the inflammation, and cause suppuration, or may pierce the bowel. But that is not all. Who would suppose that so light an article as arrowroot, or maizena could do mischief? Yet it may, for typhoid suppresses the flow of the saliva, as well as the secretions of other glands, the function of which is to convert starch into sugar, and consequently the undigested starch of all the foods just mentioned forms concrete masses which are a source of great danger at the critical point. Many fatal cases have occurred in this way. The patient has possibly got past the fever stage, and may have a good appetite, or even be so far on as to go out, and he sees no reason why he should not eat as usual, and he does so, but owing to the bowel being still in an unsafe or dangerous state at the critical point, a fatal mischief is done. Cases are known where the patient almost immediately became worse on receiving ordinary food. Had he or his friends known the true state of the case, or had it been explained to them in general terms so as not to create needless apprehensions, these things had never happened.

The African type of typhoid is usually accompanied by chest and liver complications, and the former requires immediate attention, as it frequently is the more dangerous part of the disease. The congestion and inflammation in the lungs is commonly treated by applying a bag of hot bran and renewing it repeatedly till the inflammation is reduced. The bran is heated in an iron pot, and is slightly moistened to prevent its being singed, otherwise it is quite dry.

RHEUMATIC FEVER.

Salix Capensis—Cape, River, or *Native Willow*—Kaffir, *um-Gcunube.*

The Native Willow is so well known as to need no description. Its leaves are small, delicate, and intensely bitter, compared with those of the Weeping Willow. The bark of the trunk is rough and deeply furrowed. *Salicin,* a glucoside, which is obtained from the tender shoots, has been employed time out of mind by the Natives, especially the Hottentots, in the cure of rheumatic fever. It prevents the malady from attacking the heart, and it reduces fever. Its place in the pharmacopœia, chiefly in the form of salicylate of soda, is now established. Though not so strong as salicylic acid, salicin is less irritant and not so depressing. This glucoside can be shown in the form of white needle-like crystals. It is found to be highly soluble in boiling water, requiring of that one part only, while of cold water 28 parts are necessary, of alcohol 60 parts, and in ether it is insoluble. Rheumatic fever frequently leaves behind it a chronic rheumatism, and a weakness of the heart and other involuntary muscles. This can be removed by a tincture of *Bulbine, Rooi wortel* (See Blood purifiers), which purifies the blood from lactic acid, and prevents a deposit which weakens the involuntary muscles. Like salicin this is depressing, and the dose at first should therefore not exceed 10 minims a day, the strength of the tincture being determined by putting one drachm of the dried tuber to each fluid ounce of the solvent.

The officinal willow from which salicin is procured is *Salix alba*. The Cape Willow is at least as good, and salicin could easily be prepared in this country.

INFLUENZA.

Eucalyptus globulus—Blue-gum.
Artemisia Afra, Jacq.—*Wormwood.*

Epidemic Influenza (*la grippe*), is a highly infectious disease, and is very different from what is called an influenza cold, though they have certain symptoms in common, and in some respects are treated in the same manner. One of the best things for warding off epidemic Influenza, and also for use in it, is ammoniated tincture of quinine. This is not always within reach, and there is a plant remedy in use, perhaps not much inferior to that.

For taking internally, from three to five blue-gum leaves are boiled slightly and a tablespoonful is administered twice a day with an interval between. The boiling should be *slight* so as not to expel the essential oil (eucalyptol) on which the virtue depends. An infusion made by pouring boiling water on the leaves after bruising them would also serve.

Besides this, the blue-gum leaves have another use. Influenza is accompanied or followed by inflammation in the lungs, with great pain in the chest and difficulty in breathing. This is successfully treated by slightly boiling a quantity of blue-gum leaves, and putting the hot liquid into a jar or jug. The patient is made to sit up in bed, and after being completely covered with a blanket to enclose his head also, he inhales the steam from the jar. This induces perspiration and gives great relief, and it has a decided effect in subduing inflammation. If used at night the inhalation induces sleep.

Wormwood is sometimes mixed with the blue-gum leaves for both external and internal use, and it is also employed for both purposes alone, though in epidemic Influenza blue-gum leaves should not be left out. Epidemic Influenza is an insidious disease, and there is great danger after it in getting up, and much more in going out too soon. Half the fatal cases have arisen from a relapse occasioned by a chill after appparent recovery.

CHAPTER XIII.

PLANTS FOR COLDS AND COUGHS.

Monsonia ovata—Hottentot, *Nceta*—Kaffir, *i-Gqita*.
Lichtensteinia interrupta, E. Mey.—Kaffir, *um-Bungashe*.
Eucalyptus globulus—*Blue-gum*.
Artemisia Afra, Jacq.—*Wormwood*—Kaffir, *um-Hlonyane*.
Pelargonium ramosissimum, Willd.
Solanum Capense, Thunb.—Kaffir, *um-Tumana*.
Helichrysum appendiculatum, Less.—Kaffir, *in-Dlebe ye-mvu*, *Sheep's ear*.
Lippia asperifolia. Rich.—Kaffir, *in-Zinziniba*.
Clematis brachiata, Thunb.—*Traveller's joy*—Kaffir, *i-Tyolo*.
Pallaea hastata.
Panicum sanguinale.
Chloris compressa, Nees.—Kaffir, *u-Madolwana*.
Ranunculus Capensis, and *R. pinnatus*.
Schistostephium flabelliforme, Less.—Kaffir, *isi-Petshane*.
Leonotis Leonurus—*Red dagga*.

Monsonia ovata—Hottentot, *Nceta* or *Geita*—Kaffir, *i-Gqita*.

This plant of the Order Geraniaceae is brought forward by Dr. Pappe for dysentery, its most important use. It is employed for several purposes besides, and a short description will be of advantage for its identification. Its five

H

petals are pale white with purplish streaks, very thin and semitransparent. The flowers are an inch and a half in diameter, and open out so as to lie quite flat in bright sunshine, but close up in the afternoon. The leaves are ovate, crenate, veined, three-fourths of an inch long; the flower-stalk has two bracts in the middle, and one flower—a variety has two. The whole plant is overspread with a minute pubescence, besides which the stalks, sepals, and midribs of the leaves are covered with extremely fine hairs $\frac{1}{8}$ inch long.

For colds and inflammation of the chest, the Hottentots have recourse to this plant, and make a tea of it. They collect and dry it in summer, as it dies down in winter to the root which is perennial.

The fancy that this plant owes the whole of its virtue to mere astringency is erroneous, for who in his senses would employ an astringent for a cold, when a laxative would be more to the purpose! The whole of the Geraniaceae have a sedative property running through the Order, and they have a degree of astringency, much more pronounced in some genera and species than in others. They all have an aromatic odour, varying much in character and in intensity in the different genera as well as species, though with a sufficient resemblance to afford a natural means of identification.

Lichtensteinia interrupta, E. Mey.—Kaffir, *um-Bungashe*.

An umbelliferous plant with leaves lying flat on the ground, much like carrot leaves, and a stem 20—30 inches high with an umbel of small white flowers like those of this Family. The leaf-stalks are short, flat above, rounded beneath, each terminating in three much divided leaves, the middle one largest. Each leaf is pinnate, winged between the pinnae which are farther cut, and the two lateral leaves have a pinnatifid leaflet attached to them. The bark of the root is black, and the root has the taste characteristic of the umbellifers.

The root of this plant has a considerable reputation among the Kaffirs and Basutos for curing colds, and is supposed to do so immediately. Whatever may be the truth in regard to this, it certainly has the power of giving an immediate headache. Like some other umbellifers this is a mischievous plant, and should be used with great caution. The usual way to prepare it is to boil a root! in milk, but five grains is quite enough.

Eucalyptus globulus—Blue-gum.
Artemisia Afra, Jacq.—*Wormwood*—Kaffir, *um-Hlonyane.*

Besides its use as a prophylactic from malaria, Blue-gum is valuable in various forms of chest complaint. Wormwood, of which there is only one Cape species, is employed similarly. Its uses, except this, are given by Dr. Pappe. A decoction, or other preparation, of blue-gum leaves and of wormwood mixed, or of either alone, is taken for a common cold, for an influenza cold, or for catarrh. A common use of wormwood for a cough with febrile symptoms is to administer a decoction sweetened with sugar or honey—and this especially with children.

A more important use is to inhale the steam from a

strong decoction of the leaves of both blue-gum and wormwood, or of either, while a person in bed is covered over with a blanket. This causes profuse perspiration and and gives immediate relief.

For colds, the Hottentots make use of *Helichrysum nudiflorum*, Less.—Kaffir, *i-colocolo*.

Pelargonium ramosissimum, Willd.

This Pelargonium is very unlike the common species of the genus. The leaves are pinnately parted with very short pinnae still farther divided, rough, and on hairy leaf-stalks. The narrow petals have long claws. From its peculiar smell probably, as well as its appearance, the plant is styled *dassie buchu*, though it has no relation whatever to the Buchu family. It grows in the Divisions of Burghersdorp, Middleburg, and Beaufort West.

This plant is used by the natives for colds; but it has been employed with advantage in threatened consumption for its sedative effect on the entire mucous membrane, and as a nerve tonic. An alcoholic tincture is preferable to a preparation with water, which is apt to upset weak stomachs.

Solanum Capense, Thunb.—Kaffir, *um-Tumana*,

(See DISTEMPER.) The root is used for a cough.

Withania somnifera, Dun.—Kaffir, *ubu-Vumba*.

(See SORES, Animal.) A decoction of the bark of the root is used for asthma. A decoction of the root-bark of this and of *um-Tumana*, drunk hot, is used for other chest complaints.

Helichrysum appendiculatum, Less.—Kaffir, *in-Dlebe yemvu,* Sheep's ear.

The root leaves of this plant, lying flat on the ground, both in shape and from their woolliness much resemble a sheep's ear. The stem is woolly, with many oblong pointed leaves, and a head of many flowers.

The leaves are used for chest complaint, and for that are sometimes eaten raw.

Lippia asperifolia, Rich.—Kaffir, *in-Zinziniba.*

This is a shrub, 3—4 feet high, with leaves veined and rugose resembling those of Red Dagga, only much smaller, having an extremely strong and peculiar odour. The flowers are small, cream-coloured, forming a head. Corolla tubular with a spreading limb, 2-labiate, lower lip 3-fid, stamens 4, two longer.

A decoction of the leaves, mixed with a decoction of wormwood, is used in colds—perhaps rather in a sort of low feverish inflammation in the lungs, common among the natives. *In-zinziniba* is also made use of to prevent inflammation in fever, influenza, and measles. This shrub is found in profuse quantities around King William's Town.

Clematis brachiata, Thunb.—*Traveller's joy*—Kaffir, *i-Tyolo*

(See BOTS.) If the stems of *Clematis* are broken and bruised, and placed under the nostrils, when the air is strongly drawn in, the volatile principle they give out has a pungency like smelling-salts, and will induce sneezing. This is done to remove the stuffed condition of the nostrils induced by a cold.

Pellæa hastata—*Hard fern.*

The leaves of this fern, which is very variable in form, are smoked for asthma. By some it is referred to the genus *Pteris;* by others to *Allosorus*.

Panicum sanguinale.

This is a tall grass, with a stalk 3—3½ feet high, and four spikes forming a terminal simple umbel.

A decoction is given for a cough in children. It acts by inducing vomiting.

Chloris compressa, Nees—Kaffir, *u-Madolwana* (dimin. of *i-dolo,* knee).

The spikes of this grass are digitate, with spikelets sessile on one side of a common axis. The plant is extremely hairy all over.

The grass, or its roots are boiled to make a bath for a cold, and also for rheumatism.

Ranunculus Capensis, and R. *pinnatus.*

(See STOMACH.) For bad cough and sore throat, the roots of *Ranunculus* and those of *Helichrysum nudiflorum* are boiled in sweet milk. In cases of a chill from bathing after being heated, the leaves of *Ranunculus* are bruised in water, and this is applied over the body. The acrid juice of this plant may have the virtue of restoring the tone to the skin. It was the best thing the Kaffirs had.

It is perhaps hardly known that the one effective substance for this purpose is acetic acid.

Schistostephium flabelliforme Less.—Kaffir, *isi-Petshane*.

This composite grows in high and moist situations. It is plentiful on the Katberg and in Tembuland and elsewhere. The heads of the flowers are in a corymb, numerous, yellow. The leaves and stems are silvery gray, covered with close-pressed silky hairs. The leaves in form are wedge like at the base, deeply crenate or 5—9 lobed opposite the base.

The plant is aromatic and bitter. An infusion is used for a cough. This is one of the best of the so called teas, for that purpose.

Leonotis leonurus—Red dagga.

(See SNAKE-BITE.) It is supposed that the medical virtues of this plant have by no means been exhausted. Rev. W. S. Davis of Clarkebury, than whom none have better opportunities of testing the thing, states that he administers a tincture made from the flowers for coughs and chest affections, giving in a little water from 5 to 10 drops as a dose for an adult; and as much as a tea-spoonful for severe headache; for a nervous headache it is of great benefit.

CHAPTER XIV.

REMEDIES FOR TAPEWORM.

Aloe tenuior, Haw.—Kaffir, *i-Kalana.*
Leonotis leonurus—Red Dagga—Kaffir, *um-Fincafincane.*
Rumex Eckloni—Smaller Dock—Kaffir, *i-Dolo lenkonyana* (calf's knee).
Oxalis Smithii, Sond.—*Sorrel*—Kaffir, generic name *um-Muncwane.*
Agrimonia Eupatoria, Lin., var. *Capensis—Agrimony*—Kaffir, *in-Nyinga.*
Sanseviera thyrsiflora—Kaffir, *isi-Kolokoto.*

The common mode of expelling tape-worms proceeds on the idea of poisoning them with a drug, taken on an empty stomach, and then removing them by a purge. The oil of Male Fern is the most efficacious of the poisons for tapeworm; *Kousso,* the dried flowers of *Brigera anthelmintica,* both purgative and poisonous, is also employed, and castor-oil is the best aperient. Male Fern often fails when used alone, for though the segments may come off, the head which is hooked to the mucous membrane may not imbibe the poison, and the worm will grow again. Thirty drops of chloroform are therefore now added to the usual dose of Male Fern for an adult, and that stupefies the tape-worm, so that it relaxes its hold and is killed by the drug. The dose is taken in the morning, on the presumption that all food in process of digestion has after the fast over night passed on from where the head of the tape-worm is lodged, which is assumed to be the stomach. This tacit assumption in the majority of cases is erroneous, for though occasionally the head is found in the stomach, the upper intestine is the place of attachment usually. In persons with weak action of the digestive organs the common method frequently fails. Skilful physicians have accordingly adopted the method of clearing the way for the Male Fern by giving a prior dose of castor-oil, and only after it has operated proceeding in the way stated.

Aloe tenuior, Haw.—Kaffir, *i-Kalana*.

The prevalence of tape-worm *(i-palo)* among the natives is shown in the number of remedies they employ for it. So much depends on the mode of using a remedy by fasting beforehand with the subsequent use of a purgative, that a second class remedy properly taken may be more effectual than a first class one used improperly. The advantage of knowing various remedies is, that one succeeds when another has failed, and in fact every remedy for this malady is liable to fail occasionally.

I-Kalana is a small aloe with a long, trailing, jointed stem about the thickness of a finger. The leaves are a foot long, an inch broad at the widest part, tapering, *serrated at the edges*, with fine teeth. The flowers which are at the top of the flower stalk are tubular, an inch long, $\frac{1}{6}$ inch wide, *light yellow*.

This is perhaps the most notable of the purely Kaffir remedies for tape-worm. The root is the part used, and its special virtue is believed to lie in its certainty, even when other remedies have failed; but the time it may take is uncertain. Like *kousso* it is both purgative, and poisonous to tape-worms. Sometimes it effects a perfect expulsion of the tape-worm at once; in other cases it may take a week or more; but to compensate for this, the doses may be repeated indefinitely without apparently doing any injury. The other remedies are more or less noxious, and require a rather nice adjustment to poison the tape-worm without poisoning the patient. If they fail, it becomes dangerous to repeat them. The way to use *i-kalana* is to make a decoction of a small quantity of the roots. It would be specially suited for children, though not for them only.

Leonotis leonurus—Red dagga—Kaffir, *um-Fincafincane*.

(See SNAKE-BITE.) An Inspector in the Agricultural Department had twice made use of the root of Male Fern for Tape-worm, but though it had removed the segments, the head with the symptoms of malaise remained, and the tape-worm grew again. When out hunting he happened to suck the bitter-sweet flowers of Red dagga, and soon afterwards found that the tape-worm was gone, as every symptom disappeared. He attributed that to the juice of the flowers taken on an empty stomach, as he knew of no other cause, and he was subsequently assured that Red dagga was an infallible cure for tape-worm. His informant mentioned a case in proof. He had been travelling with a nephew, and noticing that he looked ill, ascertained that tape-worm was the cause. He accordingly bruised a small quantity of Red dagga leaves and poured boiling water on them and gave him a cupful. It cured him effectually.

The flowers can be obtained only in March and April, but a preparation of the leaves, which may be sweetened a little, or of the dried flowers, is always available. In cases where Male Fern has failed, and when more or stronger doses cannot be administered without danger, Red dagga would probably prove a good substitute. It might be advisable in using it to add 30 drops of chloroform to the proper dose for an adult, on the same principle as is done with the oil of Male Fern. *Klip dagga (Leonotis ovata)* would serve instead of Red dagga.

Rumex Eckloni—Smaller Dock—Kaffir, *i-Dolo lenkonyana* (calf's knee).

This dock is found in moist places, and usually forms a mass with tangled roots and prostrate stems. The leaves may be about 6 inches in length, and $1\frac{1}{4}$ in breadth, but the size of the plant varies with the situation.

One would hardly imagine a weed of this sort to be good for anything. However, the roots are boiled in sweet milk, and this is administered for tape-worm. Occasionally the roots are simply chewed and the saliva swallowed.

Oxalis Smithii, Sond.—*Sorrel*—Kaffir, generic name *um-Muncwane*.

This sorrel has no stem, or a very short one, and is smooth. The leaves are stalked, with two-lobed leaflets, which are hollow-dotted and frequently brown beneath. The flowers are white with a yellow throat. The plant is plentiful near Lovedale. Some of the varieties found elsewhere have blueish or lilac flowers.

The bulb of this oxalis is called *uzoto* or *inkolwane*. It is ovate, brownish, and is the part used, not the cylindrical transparent portion into which the root expands. The bulbs are dried and ground to a powder, a handful of which is given in a cup of hot sweet milk, or of cold sour milk. It acts immediately and expels the body of the tape-worm, but not always the head. There appear to be other species of Oxalis, the bulbs of which serve the same purpose.

Agrimonia Eupatoria, Lin., var. *Capensis*, Harv.—*Agrimony*—Kaffir, *in-Nyinga*.

Agrimony is one of the most widely distributed plants. It is found with variations in Europe, Asia, N. America, and South America. The leaves are compound, with 3 or 4 pairs of leaflets, and a terminal one. The leaflets are coarsely toothed, and hairy beneath. The plant has a tall spike of yellow flowers. It is rather a coarsely grown plant in this country, and the seed with its hooked bristles is almost as mischievous in the wool of sheep and in the hair of angora goats as the Australian bur-weed.

Agrimony is used in England to make a stomachic tea, and the old Hottentot women are said to use it for the same purpose. It has an aromatic smell and a bitter taste. The Kaffirs employ it for the expulsion of tape-worm, and some who have it take a course of this remedy every year to bring off the body, though it fails to dislodge the head. The mode of using it is to administer a paste of the leaves in sour milk—not in sweet milk—or the same with the roots, only a less quantity. Agrimony is a very poor remedy for tape-worm.

Sanseviera thyrsiflora—Kaffir, *isi-Kolokoto*.

This plant is frequently to be seen beneath trees and in thickets, with its sword-shaped, leathery leaves, with a red border, and zig-zag white markings. Its root is given by Dr. Pappe as used for piles. The Kaffirs employ a decoction of the rootstock to expel all kinds of worms—tape-worms, thread-worms, and red-worms (intshulube). An experienced native declares it to be very efficacious.

The ordinary mode is to chew a piece of the root two inches long, and swallow the juice. For piles this must be done regularly over a period, otherwise it will be of no use.

There are other remedies for tape-worm. One of them is a decoction of a mixture of the roots of *um-Nukambiba* (Myaris inæqualis—Limoen hout), of *um-Nunguma-bele* (Paarde praam), and of *um-Nquma* (Olive)—and that is said to effect an entire expulsion. The use of *Pumpkin seeds* is also known, 30 seeds slightly roasted, are chewed and swallowed on a perfectly empty stomach—and ten minutes after, a strong dose of castor oil. There is also the *Pomegranate*; a handful of the bark of the roots is boiled an hour in water, and a half tumbler is taken after a twenty-four hours fast. There is nothing new in the last remedies, unless it be in the mode of using them.

CHAPTER XV.

PLANTS EMPLOYED IN OPHTHALMIA.

Lantana salviaefolia, Jacq.—Kaffir, *u-Tywala bentaka*, or *Bird's brandy*.

Hippobromus alata, E. and Z.—Kaffir, *u-Lwatile*—Horse-wood.

Chaenostoma rotundifolium.

Scabiosa Columbaria—*Scabious*—Kaffir, *i-Yeza lumehlo*.

Senecio deltoides, Less.

Urtica—*The nettle*—Kaffir, generic name *i-Rau*.

Ophthalmia is an inflammation in the mucous membrane (the conjunctiva), which lines the eyelids and extends over the eyeball. There is a sort of it very common, which is caused by some poison-germ or parasite, and is infectious. It is found also in cattle, sheep, and dogs, beginning with a watery running, and ending with a bleared eyeball and total blindness. The Kaffirs employ for this sort the fresh juice of the medicinal Aloe (*Aloe ferox*), or that of *Padde k!auw*. Repeated washing with a mild lotion of corrosive sublimate, 1 grain to 8 fluid oz. of water, would be more to the purpose, and the use of a salve to prevent the eyelids from sticking when closed at night.

These applications are made to arrest the inflammation before it issues in a bleared blueish eyeball. It is stated, however, by Major Boyes, a Resident Magistrate, that he has cured even this in horses. The mode he adopted was to reduce the backbone of the cuttle fish, found on the sea beach, to an impalpable powder, and blow it into the eye with a quill, repeating that every second day, until the eye clears again, and sight is restored. The blueish opaqueness for which this is a remedy might arise from a blow, or from other causes, and the cure would apply equally to other animals besides horses.

Lantana salviaefolia, Jacq.—Kaffir, *u-Tywala bentaka*, or *Bird's brandy*.

This is a bushy plant, frequently climbing, but low and spreading when standing alone. It is recognizable by its heads of small pink flowers with a white throat, varying in number, 2-labiate, upper lip slightly cleft, lower 3-lobed; when in fruit, by its clusters of small drupes, larger than those of the bramble, turning purple in ripening. The leaves, $1\frac{1}{4}$ inch by $\frac{3}{4}$ inch, are ovate, pointed, regularly serrated, with deep veins longitudinal and transverse, covered with soft pressed-down hairs above, and downy beneath.

A lotion is made from this plant for the cure of ophthalmia. It derives its Kaffir name from its fruit having the repute of intoxicating birds. An infusion of the fresh leaves is the best preparation, but they do not lose their virtue when dried, though some of the strength is lost. The value of this plant is in cases of infectious ophthalmia, and when bacteria and poison germs have been introduced; and the application produces at first burning pain. In cases where the eyes are inflamed from cold, or some such cause, its application is purely mischievous. One experienced native herb-doctor reduces the leaves and stem to a paste and applies it to bad sores. This implies a germ-killing virtue. A skilled medical practitioner who had been experimenting with this plant, found curiously enough that one or two tea-spoonfuls of an infusion of the leaves, administered every two or three hours, produced a marked benefit in cases of incipient bronchial affections.

Hippobromus alata, E. and Z.—Kaffir, *u-Lwatile—Horse-wood.*

This is a forest tree, common in Kaffraria. The flowers are small, with 5 petals and 5 sepals. The leaves are compound, with the common leafstalk downy and winged between the leaflets, of which there are usually five pairs, imperfectly opposite, with a terminal one. The leaflets are sessile, deeply toothed, leathery, smooth, with margin reflexed, base of the leaflets wedge shaped. The fruit is the size of a large pea. The leaves are inflammable from the presence of a resinous or oily substance. The wood has a peculiar smell, hence the name.

For sore eyes, the leaves are reduced to a paste and the juice is squeezed into the eye. This is also done with animals. Another way is to chew the leaves and put the saliva into the eye. This plant is also resorted to when there is a thickening in the cornea, commonly called a white spot in the eye ; but its virtue in that is very doubtful.

Chaenostoma rotundifolium.

This is a small plant, with a yellow salver-shaped corolla,

calyx 5-parted, four stamens, and very small round leaves. The leaves and stems are pounded, and a few drops of the juice are used for sore eyes. This remedy is esteemed by the natives a good one.

*Scabiosa Columbaria—Scabious—*Kaffir, *i-Yeza lamehlo.*

The flowerets of Scabiosa form a globose head, somewhat flattened above. Each has a 5-cleft corolla and 4 stamens, and a calyx ending in 5-bristles. This species varies extremely in the characters of the leaves and in the colours of the flowers, which are white in some localities, and blue in others, as also in the size of the head.

The root of one species, *Devil's-bit Scabious*, had once a repute in England for curing scab and some other maladies. It has a use among the Kaffirs as an eye medicine. Any of the modes of preparation will do.

Senecio deltoides, Less.

This is a climber with a yellow composite flower, and triangular-hastate, dentate, smooth leaves, found trailing over and covering hedges. A paste of the leaves is resorted to for sore eyes, but it is hardly worth anything.

*Urtica—The nettle—*Kaffir, generic name *i-Rau.*

A leaf-paste of the small native species with tender leaves, is used for sore eyes which are red all over.

CHAPTER XVI.

PLANTS USED FOR DIARRHŒA AND DYSENTERY—APERIENTS.

Dysentery differs from diarrhœa in being attended by inflammation or fever, and the discharges are mixed with blood and fœtid matter. When diarrhœa proceeds from a highly congested state of the colon, it is accompanied by straining and a tendency to frequent motions of the bowels, and this form is popularly called dysentery or dysenteric diarrhœa from those symptoms. As these maladies proceed from many different causes, and commonly enough involve complications, it cannot be supposed that a simple drug can be relied on to cure them. At the same time singular benefit has often been derived from certain plant substances, when the usual course of medicine has failed, as if they aid the curative powers of nature to rally and overcome the disease.

Pelargonium reniforme, Curt.—Dutch, *Rabassam*, Vulg. *Rabas*—Kaffir, *i-Yeza lezikali*.
Sutherlandia frutescens, R. Br.—Dutch *Kanker bos*.
Rubia petiolaris, DC.—Dutch, *Rooi houtje*.
Solanum Capense, Thunb.—Kaffir, *um-Tumana*.
Cassia mimosoides, Lin.—Kaffir, *um-Ngana*.

Pelargonium reniforme, Curt.—Dutch, *Rabassam*, Vulg. *Rabas*—Kaffir, *i-Yeza lezikali*.

This is a very recognizable species of Pelargonium from the leaves when mature being silvery all over owing to a short pubescence. They are kidney-shaped, in some cases ovate, and cordate at the base, lobed or crenate, velvety, above, cottony and with very prominent nerves beneath, and they are on long stalks. There are two varieties, one with rose purple flowers with a dark-red spot and streaks at the base of the two upper petals; the other with flowers of a dark port-wine colour. Whether with good reason or not, the latter is the more highly esteemed. The root is of considerable size, and may be 3 or 4 inches long and an inch in diameter at the widest point. It does not grow in the sour veldt, nor in very dry places, and it seems to prefer a soil of crumbling rock.

This species is more astringent than *Monsonia ovata*, and it is alleged to be better suited for dysentery, while the latter is rather for diarrhœa. A Resident Magistrate in the Transkei was attacked with dysentery, and was twice entirely given up by the doctors; but each time he was cured with the root of this Pelargonium, and the root of i-Tshongwe *(Xysmalobium lapathifolium,* which see) which probably dealt with a complication. The Rev. Arthur J. Lennard, who as a missionary is familiar with the treatment of disease, as well as skilled in medicinal plants, mentions a case which shows the value of this Pelargonium in dysenteric diarrhœa. He says, "A man in my employment was in the doctor's hands for about two months without any apparent benefit, and then the disease was mastered in four days by his using this remedy. It is prepared in a simple manner. Usually the root is cut up very fine or bruised, and then boiled in milk for a considerable time. The dose as usual is uncertain." Another preparation is to remove the outer skin, dry the root, and reduce it to a powder, of which a tea-spoonful is administered in a cup of warm milk. *Pelargonium pulverulentum* (See MISCELLANEOUS), plentiful in the mountain, and near the sea, and in moist places, where the former is not found, is employed for the same purposes.

Sutherlandia frutescens, R. Br.—Dutch, *Kanker bos.*

(See CANCER.) A government Land Surveyor, when engaged in a survey, had a severe attack of what was called dysentery, but which may rather have been dysenteric diarrhœa with intense congestion of the colon, producing the frequent straining which is a symptom of dysentery. It was probably due to receiving unsuitable food, and to being jolted on rough roads in a Cape cart. He became so weak that to his feeling a straw would have pushed him over, and he thought he would have to leave off and return home. After using other remedies without effect, he was recommended to try Sutherlandia, and so a decoction of the leaves was made. After the second dose he rallied much that he carried through the survey without difficulty. Now when he goes out, he takes with him a tincture of the leaves in a phial, and if a tendency to a return of anything similar shows itself, a tea-spoonful of the tincture removes it at once. The action of Sutherlandia in this case is probably not due to astringency.

Rubia petiolaris, D C.—Dutch, *Rooi houtje*.

This plant is found growing beneath mimosas. The leaves are in whorls and stalked, the lower somewhat cordate pointed, the upper lanceolate. The angles of the quadrangular stem, the leaf-stalks, the edges and midrib of the leaves are all furnished with prickles like teeth, which point downward. The roots are red both in the bark and within.

A decoction of the root is employed for dysentery. In bad cases this is mixed with a decoction of the roots of the following—*umtumana*.

Solanum Capense, Thunb.—Kaffir, *um-Tumana*.

(See DISTEMPER.) The roots have been used for dysentery. They are powdered and mixed with sour milk.

Punica granatum—*Pomegranate*.

As the Pomegranate has a place in the Pharmacopœia, it would be needless to refer to it here except to state a mode of using it for dysentery which is different from the ordinary mode, and is highly spoken of. An infusion, or slight decoction, of a small handful of pomegranate peel is put in a quart of new milk. To this is added a tablespoonful of French brandy, set on flame for a little; or more, if the patient is weak; and the yolk of an egg beaten up. It must be prepared fresh every day. This is taken as a drink, and acts gradually.

Cassia mimosoides, Lin.—Kaffir, *um-Nyana*.

A Leguminous plant resembling the mimosa in the form and arrangement of the leaflets on its compound leaves—hence its specific name, and its Kaffir name, a diminutive of *um-Nga* the mimosa. The leaflets are in pairs from 10 to 34, linear, in shape resembling the blade of a large clasp-knife, with the midrib near the straight edge and projecting a little at the tip, and with striæ proceeding obliquely from the midrib across the large half. The flowers are orange-yellow. The plant is plentiful at the head of the Mankazana valley near Chumie Peak, at Komgha, Main, and near King William's Town.

It has been repeatedly stated from independent sources, that this plant boiled in milk is a cure for dysentery. Had it been said—for diarrhœa, it would have been improbable, since senna is a *cassia*. Dysentery, however, is different, and is frequently occasioned by an effort to throw some poison out of the system.

The entire plant is also used for eruptions in the face.

APERIENTS.

*Euclea lanceolata—Guarri—*Dutch, *Bosch guarri—*Kaffir, *i-Yeza lokuxaxazisa.*
Euphorbia pugniformis, and *E. bupleurifolia,* Jacq.— Kaffir, *in-Kamamasane.*
*Aloe ferox—*Kaffir, *um-Hlaba.*

---

*Euclea lanceolata—Guarri—*Dutch, *Bosch guarri—*Kaffir, *i-Yeza lokuxaxazisa,* or *um-Gwali.*

This is a forest tree, found also in patches of bush. The leaves are lanceolate, leathery, margin slightly waved, scaly and of a light colour beneath. The flowers are small; fruit a one-seeded berry.

The bark of the roots is purgative. A decoction is employed, and its action is said to be rapid. The same preparation is used for biliousness.

Euphorbia pugniformis, and *Euphorbia bupleurifolia,* Jacq.—Kaffir, generic name *in-Tsema,* specific *in-Kamamasane.*

(See CANCER.) These plants are used as purgatives by taking dough of Kaffir-corn meal, and collecting the milk from them on it, about half a teaspoonful. This is then boiled along with more meal into a thin porridge, which is drunk and acts as a violent emetic. Broth is then taken which checks the vomiting, and induces severe purging. It often happens that during the action of the medicines the patient has to be held down with great force, and the limbs kept stretched out, otherwise they would be drawn together. This occurs when an overdose is given. The euphorbia milk acts like croton oil, and is not less dangerous. It is of some importance in obstinate constipation, or where people on occasions gorge themselves with food.

Aloe ferox, var. *supralaevis*—*The medicinal Aloe*—Kaffir, *um-Hlaba*.

The medicinal Aloe of the Eastern Districts with its thick glaucous green leaves, with brown prickles at the edges and tall spiked raceme of light red flowers has well known properties; but there are some things which have not been said about it. It occurs in quantity on the slopes of stony hills facing the sun. Aloes cannot be procured by cutting off the point of a leaf and allowing it to bleed, because the sap flows backwards. The leaves must be cut from the plant and suspended with the base downward over a tin or other shallow vessel. When the juice is exposed to the air for two or three days it becomes dry, and is yellow and transparent like resin; afterwards it darkens a little. It has a peculiar and not agreeable odour. The mistake of using it alone as an aperient is frequently made in this country, in which form it is irritating. It should be mixed with an equal amount of Castile soap, and the two moistened should be melted together. This makes a good simple aloetic pill. The fresh aloe juice is dropped into the eye by the Kaffirs, and also in Basutoland and Zululand, for the worst kind of ophthalmia. It may possibly have some germ-killing power, and its use to cure scab in sheep implies some power of destroying the lower forms of animal life. There are some reasons of a general kind for supposing that in this country where it grows, its use ought to be preferred to that of foreign aloes from its possessing some distinctive property suitable to the forms of maladies found in the country.. Kaffir children are fond of sucking the sweet juice of the red flowers, and when this is done to any extent, it is said to produce extreme weakness of the joints, which lasts a long time. This juice is said to be narcotic.

If a horse is infested with ticks, they will fall off after a table-spoonful of aloes has been administered. That shows its penetrating nature in going through the blood.

CHAPTER XVII.

HEADACHE.

Anemone Caffra, E. and Z.—Kaffir, *i-Yezu elimnyama*.
Ricinus communis, Lin.—Castor-oil shrub—Kaffir, *um-Hlavutwa*.
Datura Stramonium, Lin.—Kaffir, *um-Hlavutwa*—Fingo, *um-Vumbangwe*.

Anemone Caffra, E. and Z.—Kaffir, *i-Yezu elimnyama*.

This anemone is plentiful on the south side of the Katberg, and on the high parts of the mountain near Main in Tembuland. It has hard stiff leaves, usually 7-lobed, serrate with smaller teeth on some of the larger, rough and bristly at the edge and coloured with the purple which comes out on the back of the leaf. The leaf-stalks come from the rootstock, and are 3—4 inches long. The flowers are large, white, and the rootstock, is acrid and bitter, with the bark black.

For headache, the root is ground, and a pinch of the powder is used as snuff. If that does not give relief, the hairy upper part of the rootstock is lighted, and the smoke is drawn in through the nostrils for a short time, and the leaves are ground to a paste with a few drops of water, and the paste is rubbed on the part affected.

The efficacy of this remedy is spoken of with confidence, but it would depend entirely on the kind of headache. The failure of many of these specifics arises probably from using them for a purpose for which they are quite unfitted.

A skilful native doctoress, who uses this plant for curing headache in the manner stated, undertakes the treatment of madness with this and another plant *i-Yeza logezo* (remedy for madness), *Athrixia heterophylla*, Less. This plant, belonging to the Compositæ, has the lower leaves ovate, the upper linear, with revolute margin, very green and shining above, white and woolly beneath, the upper side rough with minute raised points. The flowers have a yellow disk and a pale purplish pink ray.

The mode of using the plant is to administer a decoction of the root, and a snuff is made of the dried root and also of the root of *iyeza elimnyama* together, and patients are made to snuff this till they sneeze. No doubt the madness in question is merely that which comes

HEADACHE.

from milk-fever, or from some such temporary cause.

Ricinus communis, Lin.—*Castor-oil shrub.*—Kaffir, *um-Hlavutwa.*

Datura Stramonium, Lin.—Kaffir, *um-Hlavutwa*—Fingo, *um-Vumbangwe.*

The leaves of the Castor-oil shrub are applied externally to cure headache, and are better than the next.

The leaves of Stramonium have been employed similarly, and are said to produce sweating; but this is a dangerous remedy. A boy on whom it was inadvertently tried had the pupil of one eye permanently dilated, but fortunately the natural state was restored after a week by excluding the light with a bandage. One would expect that Stramonium would have some properties allied to Belladonna, from their belonging to the same Family, the Solanaceæ. It is well known that Belladonna dilates the pupil of the eye.

CHAPTER XVIII.

TOOTHACHE—SORE THROAT—EARACHE.

TOOTHACHE.

Blepharis Capensis, and *Crabbea cirsioides*—Kaffir, *ubu-Hlungu besigcawu.*

(See SNAKE-BITE.) These are much the best of the toothache plants. They are strongly antiseptic, and will arrest decay by removing its cause. They may have some action on the nerve of the tooth. A paste of the leaves is used. The roots have the same virtue, and a tincture of the entire plants may be employed. How far these or any other plants can afford relief in toothache is a question. Toothache is connected with some irritation, nervous or mucous, in the stomach or viscera, and it is frequently occasioned by damp. Till the more remote cause is removed, a local remedy can do little. The dried leaves and roots of these plants triturated would make with aromatic chalk an excellent tooth powder from their antiseptic qualities.

Solanum Capense, Thunb,—Kaffir, *um-Tumana.*

A Solanum is easily recognized from its flower with a 5 parted corolla, lilac, purple, or white, and a central column of stamens with elongated bright yellow anthers. This species is a low trailing bush, often found growing on or beside ant-heaps, not exceeding a foot in height, with spreading branches frequently lying on the ground. It is very prickly. The leaves are lobed, about 1¼ inch long by ½ inch wide. The flowers are small and white. It bears a light-red naked berry the size of a large pea. The berry when unripe has the end next the stalk white, the other end green; thus reversing the arrangement found in some other species. A species of Solanum hardly distinguishable from this has been described under the name of *S. supinum* or *pro—*or *de-cumbens.* It may be a mere variety of *S. Capense,* but in any case they may be used for the same purpose.

There are Native experts who allege that they know a root which can make a tooth drop out. It is impossible to believe the absurd stories told about this, and it is difficult to comprehend the mode in which a root could cause it. One can understand the value of such an appliance, if it exist, in removing the stumps of decayed or broken teeth without the wrenching, the torture, or the use of gas, necessary in extraction, The root of Solanum Capense is one of the things which have some such power. A European trader who communicated the knowledge of its virtue tried it on himself, and found that it brought out the tooth he wished, but also from incautious use the one next it. The mode of using it is to powder the dried root, make a ball with moisture of the powder, and put it in the hollow tooth, or on the stump. This may require to be done repeatedly.

Lasiosiphon Meisneri—Kaffir, *isi-Dikili*. (SORES.)

When people are tortured with stings of pain from a decayed tooth, the root of *isi-Dikili* will remove the pain. Some of the cottony fibres are made up into a ball, and put into the hollow tooth. It may scorch the tonsils somewhat, but a case is known in which it removed the toothache in ten minutes.

Indigofera patens. (STOMACH.)

This Indigofera has a power to deaden pain—a character of the genus. If a portion of the root powdered is put into a tooth, it will stop the toothache.

Xanthoxylon Capense—Dutch, Paarde praam—Kaffir, *um-Nunyumabele*.

The inner bark of this tree or shrub pounded to a paste and applied to an aching tooth takes away all pain.

Besides the plants named a paste of the leaves of *Padde klauw* (SNAKE-BITE) is put into a tooth for toothache; and also the white root of *Ranunculus*. (STOMACH.)

SORE THROAT.

Brachylaena elliptica, Less.—Dutch, *Bitter blar*—Kaffir, *isi-Duli*.

This tree is a Composite with heads of numerous small flowers, and is easily recognized from its leaves which are of a very dark glossy green above, woolly and white beneath. In shape the typical leaf is three-lobed at the apex and is narrowed like a wedge from that point to the base; though the leaves are often simply obovate but very elongate. They are toothed, sinuate, or otherwise entire, at the margin. This species is found in thickets throughout the Eastern Districts. It bears some likeness to the bastard olive, but can readily be distinguished from it by the softness of its wood—it is a firestick—and by its leaves which contrast with the dull green above and gray below of that olive.

A strong decoction made from the leaves of *Bitter blar* is an important gargle for malignant sore throat. It cleans out the sores, leaving red flesh, and prepares for healing. The mouth and throat of a child were in such a state of ulceration that the doctor gave up the case. They were then washed with a strong decoction of the leaves, which cleaned out the ulcers and removed the membranous looking skin, leaving the parts red and raw. The child, soon after, wished for something to drink, and recovered rapidly.

The leaves are not poisonous, so that should a little of the decoction be swallowed, no harm comes of that. A decoction has been employed with good effect in loosening a severe cold which had taken hold of the chest.

The bark of the mimosa and that of the olive are in common use as gargles in sore throat, but are probably not equal to *bitter blar*.

Lasiosiphon linifolius, Meisn.

For the other species, see SNAKE-BITE. This species differs from the others in having longer and more pointed leaves; flowers yellow, but not bright. It is abundant on the ridges behind Lovedale and between the Swelamanzi and Nqayi valleys. The roots are not behind those of the other species in their scorching quality, though tasteless at first. They are employed by decoction, or simply by chewing, for certain forms of sore throat. Perhaps a decoction might be used with advantage as a substitute for a solution of lunar caustic as a lotion for the back of the throat. Its application is safer, and there are no after effects.

It is said that this species has been used in snake-bite; but L. Meisneri is the proper one. The roots of some species of *Gnidia*, a genus closely allied to *Lasiosiphon*, have similar blistering properties.

Padde klauw (See SNAKE-BITE.) is also used for sore throat. Either the leaves are chewed, so that the juice mixes with the saliva; or a small quantity of a decoction is taken internally. This is especially when there are small tumours in the inside of the throat.

EARACHE.

Cotyledon orbiculata, Linn.—Kaffir, *i-Pewula*.

I-Pewula is a generic name for thick-leafed plants of this class. This species has bell-shaped, fleshy, drooping, red flowers on long stalks. The whole plant in stem and branches is like the exotic scarlet geranium. Its leaves are obovate, wedge-shaped at the base, have a bloom, and a red border.

The juice of the leaves is warmed and put into the ear for earache. Some other species would do equally well.

It serves an excellent purpose in corns, as described by Dr. Pappe, and as found in common use. The skin of a broad leaf is removed, and the fleshy part is applied under a sock night and day. This renewed morning and evening quickly renders the corn soft and easily removed.

CHAPTER XIX.

STYPTICS—ITCH—WORMS—EPILEPSY.

STYPTICS.

Chenopodium vulvaria, Lin.—*A goosefoot*—Kaffir, au *im--Bikicane*.

This is a weed common in gardens and in fields. The flowers are small, greenish. In a small-grown specimen, the leaves are entire; those near the top of the twigs are ovate, pointed; the others are blunt, and are broadened near the base, contracting suddenly towards the leafstalk. In large specimens the leaves show a tendency to become rhomboidal, only long towards the point of the leaf and blunt angled at the stalk, with a sinuate margin. The leaves are covered with a blue mealiness, which appears under an eye-glass as glittering grains. The whole plant is blueish-green, the twigs reddish. It has a fœtid smell. The *Chenopodium* with rhomboidal, deeply veined, toothed, larger leaves is another garden weed, sometimes used by the Colonists as a spinage.

A paste of the leaves of *C. vulvaria* is a rather effective styptic. It is only for external application. It was used with success by a farmer to stop profuse bleeding in the case of an ox, where an ulcerous swelling had been incautiously removed.

K

Bulbine asphodeloides, Schult.—Dutch, *Wilde Capive*.

(See SCROFULA.) The juice of this plant also is said to have styptic properties—for external use. Although some of these vegetable styptics are good for something and are accessible, none of them approaches in efficacy the perchloride of iron.

Solanum Sodomaeum—Bitter apple—Kaffir, *um-Tuma*.

Solanums are easily recognised from the yellow anthers standing erect and close together so as to form a pyramid, and from the fruit which is either a naked berry or a plum. This Solanum has the corolla an inch broad, five angled, lilac with a purple streak at the lower part of the rib running from each angle. The fruit is a plum, $1\frac{1}{4}$—$1\frac{3}{4}$ inches, largest 2 inches, in diameter; when unripe, green at the stalk and white at the opposite end, the two colours crossing each other in a fingered manner; when ripe, entirely of a warm yellow. The leaves are both rugose, and rough with very short bristles; they have two or three blunt lobes on each side, the indentations nearly as large, with spines on the ribs, on both sides of the leaf. There is a species in or near the forests which might be mistaken for this from the description, but the leaves are flat, with the lobes pointed, and those at the base of the leaf are much larger. The hairs and the leaves are soft, and the spines slender. In the plum, when unripe, the colours are reversed, the white end being at the stalk; when ripe, it is of a whitish yellow, and is smaller than the former.

Before European remedies were brought within their

reach, the Kaffirs resorted to *Solanum Sodomaeum,* a species of the genus *um-Tuma,* for itch (u-kwekwe) and also for scab. They employed a paste of the leaves and also the juice of the plum, applied externally. The same was used for scab in sheep. Some of the Solanums are bacteria killers; others destroy parasites and the lower forms of animal life. This Solanum is said to be sometimes used for sores on the backs of horses. Its virtue would depend on the nature of the sore.

WORMS.

Hibiscus Trionum, Lin.—Kaffir, *i-Ycza lentshulube.*

This Hibiscus is an annual and is common. It is hairy, with leaves varying excessively in form. The corolla is primrose yellow with a dark port wine coloured centre. An inflated many-ribbed calyx, bladder-like after flowering, is distinctive of this species.

It is employed as a remedy for red worms—*intshulube.*

For red worms, thread worms, and for tape-worm, the Kaffirs also use *isi-kolokoto*—*Sanseviera thyrsiflora,* Thunb. —described by Pappe as used in piles. A decoction of the root-stock is the preparation. There is a larger forest kind called *isi-kolokoto sehlati.*

EPILEPSY.

Exomis axyrioides, Fenzl.

A helpless epileptic had spent on doctors all he had to spend, with no benefit. He was recommended to try a

Hottentot remedy, the leaves of this low shrub, which the Dutch call *Honde bos*. The preparation is a decoction in milk of a small handful of the leaves, a tablespoonful of which is taken for a few days thrice a day immediately after meals. Water will not suit, as a water decoction produced stupor. The result of the treatment was that the man recovered, and epilepsy did not return. The shrub grows on a saline soil and is glaucous in appearance. One can hardly fancy such a worthless weed to be good for anything; but the facts remain as stated.

CHAPTER XX.

REMEDIES FOR RINGWORM—KIDNEY DISORDER—LUMBAGO.

RINGWORM.

Aloe saponaria, or *latifolia* of Haw.—*White spotted Aloe* —Kaffir, *in-Gcelwane*.
Solanum nigrum, Lin.—*Nightshade*—Kaffir, *um-Sobo*.
Withania somnifera, Dun.—Kaffir, *ubu-Vumba*

Before anything is used to kill the fungoid germ which causes ringworm, it is necessary to wash the part affected very thoroughly so as to remove everything which would hinder the substance employed from reaching the germs.

Aloe saponaria—White-spotted Aloe—Kaffir, *in-Gce-lwane.*

For a notice of the plant see under WOUNDS. The leaf is cut open and applied, and the yellow juice from the base of the leaf should also be rubbed in. This remedy is said to be very efficacious, and to remove ringworm so that it will not return.

Solanum nigrum, Lin.—*Nightshade*—Kaffir, *um-Sobo.*

This Solanum is well known growing as a weed in gardens, and in cultivated fields where the soil is rich. It has small white flowers, rather large ovate crenate leaves. The berries are black when ripe, and are sometimes eaten by children under the name of *um-Sobosobo.* For ringworm, a paste of the green berries is used.

Withania somnifera, Dun.—Kaffir, *ubu-Vumba.*

(See SORES—Animal.) The green berries of this plant are bruised and rubbed in for Ringworm. They effect a cure very quickly.

In-Tsema.

There is a large globular bulb, the size a boy's head, the milky juice of which is sometimes used for Ringworm.

KIDNEY DISORDERS.

Hermannia candicans, Ait.
Eriosema salignum, E. Mey.—Kaffir, *um-Fisi.*

Hermannia candicans.

The petals of this plant are spirally twisted in aestivation, five, yellow. The leaves are oblong ovate, obtuse, waved in outline as well as toothed, woolly above, more so below, stalked. It is plentiful near Lovedale and in Kat River.

A decoction of the roots is used for dysuria. It is blue when boiled in an iron vessel and greenish in a tin, and becomes starchy when cold.

Eriosema Salignum, E. Mey.—Kaffir, um-Fisi.

The stems, flower and leaf-stalks of this leguminous plant are covered with soft hairs. The leaflets of the compound leaf are three, oblong, pointed, pilose above, silky, and white with a blueish effect, beneath. The flowers are orange. A small amount of a pink secretion is found below the bark of the root.

A decoction of the root is of service for scanty urine. For this purpose it is not considered quite so good as the previous plant.

Solanum Capense or *Supinum*—Kaffir, *um-Tumana.*
Petroselinum sativum—Common *Parsley.*

(See TOOTHACHE.) The root of this Solanum is declared

to be a specific for dysuria. The dose is 10 grains of the dried root powdered, and it is said to act almost immediately.

Probably the properties of Parsley in dysuria are little known. There occurred a case of retention with frequent micturition, which lapsed into entire stoppage of the urethra from inflammatory stricture. It was found impossible to pass in a catheter, and as the doctor had no resource, the case became dangerous. A nurse suggested administering a strong infusion, made with boiling water, from the roots of parsley—the leaves however were taken as roots were not obtainable. On the infusion being drunk, it took effect in a few minutes, and the inflammation also passed away and did not return.

It is said that an infusion of the root, or of both it and the leaves, of parsley is sometimes effective in removing gravel.

LUMBAGO.

Bulbine latifolia—Kaffir, an *in-Gcelwane*—Dutch, *Rooi wortel*.

The Kaffir name is given from the plant resembling an Aloe. The leaves are close about the root-stock, broad at the base and tapering to a point, embracing, without prickles, but with a very narrow border. The flower-stalk is 12—20 inches high, with a spiked raceme of bright yellow flowers, perianth 6-parted, stamens bearded at the top. The rootstock is orange-yellow, the older parts redder, and it yields a beautiful carmine tincture. The tuber was put forward by Mr. C. L. Stretch as efficacious in lumbago.

Zizyphus mucronata, Willd.—*The Wait-a-bit thorn-tree—* Kaffir, *um-Pafa.*

(SEE SCROFULA.) A decoction of the root of this tree is also used for Lumbago.

CHAPTER XXI.

CANCER.

Euphorbia—Kaffir, *um-Hlonhlo.*
Euphorbia pugniformis—Kaffir, generic name, *in-Tsema*
—specific, *in-Kamamasane.*
Euphorbia bupleurifolia, Jacq.—Kaffir, same as last.
Sutherlandia frutescens, R. Br.

The milk of the *Euphorbias* named above, if it has any real efficacy, must be supposed both to kill the poison germs it reaches by local application, and also to destroy the fungoid growth and cause its removal by suppuration. It cannot, however, enter into the blood and kill the germs there. This is a radical defect. Still, it is by no means improbable that a remedy for cancer may be found among the *Euphorbiaceae,* capable of being administered internally to kill the germs, and there are various germ-killing plants belonging to this Family, fitted for internal use.

The milk of the common *Euphorbia* tree is well known for its blistering properties. Equal parts of the milk and of turpentine are taken, and to one part of the mixture two parts of sweet oil are added. Care must be taken in using the milk of the euphorbia, as it eats into the flesh, especially with some persons. It is a good substitute for lunar caustic; and it has been used with effect in gangrenous sores with spreading roots where after some length of time it appeared to kill the ulcer, and then the sore healed in the natural way.

Euphorbia pugniformis—Kaffir, *in-Kamamasane.*

Is cone shaped, flat at the top, breadth 3—4 inches, length about the same. The top which is level with the ground is covered with protuberances, which become large in a regular manner from the centre outwards, and are spirally arranged. Those on the outside assume a finger-like form, in one or more rows, and are crowned with a ring of bright yellow flowers.

Euphorbia bupleurifolia—Same name in Kaffir.

Is egg-shaped, below forming a pointed cone, and is usually half above ground. The upper part is covered with protuberances and is cross furrowed, with a spiral arrangement of both. It is crowned with a number of erect leaves, which are lance-shaped, and wedge-shaped at the base. They like the root are full of milk.

The generic name in Kaffir for these similar species is *in-Tsema*, but the two named are also called *in-kamamasane*. Their milk is used for cancerous sores in the same way as that of the tree Euphorbia. It is also used for painful cracked feet—*amasa*—and for some kinds of eczema, milk-crust—*um-na*.

Sutherlandia frutescens, R. Br. —Dutch, *Cancer bush*.

This shrub has been brought forward recently as a remedy for cancer, and for that reason it is noticed here. It is mentioned by Dr. Pappe in his Prodromus, who quotes Thunberg to the effect that the roots and leaves are of use in diseases of the eye. The shrub belongs to the Order *Leguminosæ*, and has compound leaves, unequally pinnate, multi-jugate, with elliptical or oblong leaflets, smooth above, slightly hoary beneath. The flowers are showy, scarlet or bright red, the legumes or seed vessels are much inflated.

There can be no reasonable doubt that Sutherlandia has been the means of curing malignant tumours, cancerous in appearance, which were firmly believed to be cancers by non-professional persons unacquainted with the distinctive marks of typical cancer. It is also certain, that employed as a blood purifier and tonic, it has delayed the progress of true cancer and much prolonged life. In view of these facts and of the confident assertions made regarding Sutherlandia, it was desirable that it should be tested in a typical case of cancer, and that was done recently by a physician of high intelligence with the result, as in some similar instances formerly, that it proved wanting though applied both externally and internally.

There is nothing in this to disprove its claim to be a plant of real importance, since it has been found efficacious in maladies which try the resources of the pharmacopoeia.

These uses will be found under the heads of Stomach disorders, Dysenteric diarrhoea, and Tonics.

CHAPTER XXII.

PLANTS CONNECTED WITH BLOOD-POISONING—CHILDREN'S &c. MEDICINES — SYPHILITIC BLOOD-POISONING — BATHS — STITCH—A RASH—BONE FRACTURE—NOTE ON SLOW ABSORPTION—ON ATROPA BELLADONNA.

BLOOD-POISONING.

The powerlessness of the usual medical appliances to arrest blood-poisoning is constantly shown. Something has been done to stop the action where it proceeds from the *milt ziek* poison, but there are cases where it arises from the simple putrefaction of animal matter, or from a product of that putrefaction, and the question is how to arrest that. In the South Sea Islands the natives poison their arrows with matter taken from the spinal region opposite the kidneys of a decaying human body. Commander Goodenongh was wounded with an arrow of this sort. He died in a few days of tetanus. Nothing could be done to save him. Cases are constantly occurring in this country of persons who are blood-poisoned in opening the body of an animal, or in cutting up meat in a decaying state. It certainly would be a triumph of discovery could plants be found capable of arresting blood-poisoning of this sort. The nearest approach to that is mentioned by Rev. W. S. Davis, of Clarkebury. "Over 80 Natives were affected with blood-poisoning through eating diseased sheep near Umtata about two years ago. 46 of them were treated by a native with the herb sent, and Leonotis leonurus, and all recovered." The plant sent to me by Mr. Davis was—*Blepharis Capensis*—Kaffir, *ubu-Hlungu besigcawu*. (See *Snake-bite*.) To show his confidence in the antidote the native drank some of the decoction himself, and ate a large quantity of the diseased meat, on seeing which the men who were lying in a dying state took the antidote and presently got up.

In the case of blood-poisoning, given under SORES, from opening an animal which died of *Spons-ziekte*, or Quarter-evil, it is a question whether the malady was caused simply by very putrid matter, or by the germ which causes a disease somewhat like *Milt-ziekte*, or Splenic fever. Perhaps the treatment mentioned here, with *Blepharis* and *Leonotis* (preferably *ovata*), would be the most suitable. It is the same as in milt-ziekte without *Monsonia*, which might properly be added.

CHILDREN'S &C. MEDICINES.

Chlorophytum comosum, Baker, or *Hartwegia comosa*, Nees—Kaffir, *u-Jejane*.

U-Jejane belongs to the Liliaceæ. It is found in moist woods under trees, plentiful in the Nqayi valley, near the Chumie, and in the lower thickets at Katberg. The flowers form a raceme on a flower-stalk 12—22 inches high, white above, green beneath, star-like, with six sepals. The leaves 6—8 inches long, 7—8 lines wide, are radical, soft, shining, slightly bordered, finely ribbed. The plant has a bundle of roots, with fleshy tubers at their extremities, cylindrical, pointed at both ends, 1¼ inch long by 3 lines wide, white and nearly transparent.

These tubers are steeped in cold water, and the infusion is given to infants on the day of birth as a purgative. It is also employed as an aperient with infants generally. This is the preferable plant, but when it cannot be had, the natives resort to *u-sikiki*, and give a cold infusion of the leaves, or as mentioned below.

Salvia scabia, Thun.—Kaffir, *u-Sikiki*.

This *Salvia* is plentiful in the Chumie valley and in the valleys running into it. The leaves are extremely rugose, the flowers blue not large. The *Salvias* seem to be used medicinally everywhere, though they are not of much consequence.

This is used as the first medicine given to infants. A paste of the leaves is given in the mother's milk.

Gazania pinnata, var. *integrifolia*—Kaffir, *um-Kwinti*—
Dutch, *Boter-bloem*.

This is one of the plants which spread out their petals in full to the midday sun. It is a Composite with a flower 2—3 inches broad. The disk is yellow; the petals of the ray are bright orange-yellow, the portion near the base of a ruby brown, shading into the yellow with a dark brown nearly black. In the middle of this ruby-coloured patch there is a small heart-shaped white spot, and each petal has a green stripe down the back. The leaves are linear, varying much in breadth, 3—4 lines, and 4—6 inches long, very white and woolly beneath, but with a green midrib, and the upper side dark green and rough with short bristles. The plant is full of a white milky juice. It is widely difused.

An infusion of the whole plant, including the roots, is used to prevent miscarriage. It is said that a decoction of the rootstock of *Bulbine latifolia*, Schult., given internally is used for the same purpose; but the authority for this is not so reliable, as that for the former.

The same was effected in an undoubted case in which all medical aid had failed, by the root of *Sanseviera thyrsiflora*—Kaffir, *isi-Kolokoto*.

To facilitate parturition by increasing the muscular action, the Natives empoly the root of *Typha latifolia*, the Reed-Mace—Kaffir, *um-Kanzi*—a marsh plant whose tall stem 6 or 7 feet high with the inflorescence at the top resembles the ramrod of a field-piece.

SYPHILITIC BLOOD-POISONING.

Cissampelos Capensis, Thunb.; *C. torulosa*; *C. Pareira*— Dutch, *Davidjes*.
Solanum melongena—Kaffir an *um-Tuma*.
Withania somnifera—Kaffir, *ubu-Vumba*.

On the strength of knowing some of the plants employed, some native empirics have made pretensions of being able to cure syphilitic disease, with the result that they effect a cure of eruptions and sores, but subsequently there breaks out elsewhere what is ascribed to a different cause altogether, though it is known by medical men to be an effect of the syphilitic poison. This has given rise to an opinion that there is no thorough Native cure for this disease. The contrary, however, is certain, and there are Native specialists who can effect a radical cure at least in the first and second stages of the disease. Cases and exceedingly bad ones could be referred to which District Surgeons and others knew to be malignant forms of the disease, and satisfied themselves that Native specialists had eradicated the disease so as not to leave a trace afterwards. The native method is to use blood-purifiers internally, and leaf-pastes and plasters externally, and the treatment may extend over a period such as two months. Whether they can do anything effective in the tertiary stage, without mercury and iodide of potassium, is very doubtful. Suppose the Native methods and appliances in this disease are not fitted to supersede those adopted in medicine, they might be employed as auxiliary, and they would afford a substitute in cases, as in those involving caries of the bone, where the use of mercury is impossible. On account of unnatural crowding in huts which favours contagion, many innocent people, children and others, are sufferers from this pernicious malady.

Cissampelos Capensis, Thunb.—*C. Torulosa*, E. Meyer— *C. Pareira*, Linn.—Dutch, *Davidjes*.

The flowers are dioecious in these plants of the Menispermaceae, axillary, whitish. The male flower has four petals confluent. They are all twining, partly climbing plants.

C. Capensis has the leaves broadly ovate—they could be called heart-shaped but that they want an indentation at the junction of the leaf-stalk, they are blunt at the apex, reticulated, and often though not always smooth. They are from $1\frac{1}{8}$ to $1\frac{1}{4}$ inch long, and 1 to $1\frac{1}{8}$ inch broad.

C. torulosa is very recognizable in the Eastern forests and thickets as a twiner with a profusion of broad kidney-shaped leaves, a full grown leaf being $1\frac{3}{4}$ inch broad by $1\frac{1}{8}$ inch long. They are not pointed.

C. Pareira has leaves between heart-shaped and kidney-shaped, pubescent, more so below. It is found in Natal.

All the species possess the distinctive properties more or less, but *C. Capensis* is much the best, and to it reference is made in what follows.

The internal use of *Davidjes* is important. An alcoholic tincture, or a preparation with brandy, will be the most suitable, making the proportion between the root finely divided and the solvent as 1 to 8; or a drachm to each fluid oz. The dose to begin with may be 10 minims in a little water, and can be given twice a day.

For external use, any of the preparations will do, such as a salve made with the root reduced to an impalpable powder; but a leaf-paste of Withania may be quite as good, or better.

Solanum melongena—Kaffir generic name, *um-Tuma*.

This Solanum is 2—4 feet high. The leaves are entire, ovate, pointed, nerved, varying in size, one half of

SYPHILITIC BLOOD-POISONING.

the leaf frequently extending down the leaf-stalk farther than the other, woolly and white beneath. The leaf-stalks and younger branches are also woolly and hoary, and the bark of the stem is of the same colour. The flowers are white and have the usual central column of yellow anthers, characteristic of the Solanums. In the unripe plum the blueish-green of the end next the stalk extends into the white of the other half in a fingered manner; when ripe it is of a bright yellow. It is an inch and two lines long by an inch and one line broad, and differs in shape from the plum of Solanum Sodomaeum which is broader than it is long. The whole plant is comparatively destitute of prickles.

For syphilitic eruptions and the other effects of the poison, a decoction of the bark of the root reduced to a powder, is administered internally; and a paste of the leaves is applied externally. This is a remedy of known efficacy, and is said to be one of the best.

Withania somnifera, Dun.—Kaffir, *ubu-Vumba*—Fingo, *u-Vimba*.

This is a plant found in gardens and in waste corners, 3 feet high, with ovate leaves. It may be readily recognized from its bright red berries, which are enclosed like the Cape gooseberry in the inflated calyx, through which they can be seen when ripe, as it is then translucent.

Like the one before it, Withania belongs to the Solanaceae, and is very widely employed in the cure of syphilitic disease, both in the Colony and right through Griqualand East to Natal. There can be no doubt of its importance especially for external use in the form of a leaf-paste, and many both Native and European regard it as far the best. A preparation from the inner bark of the root is employed internally. A guarded use is necessary, as the Solanum Family is more or less poisonous.

Besides the plants mentioned, use is made, for external application to eruptions after being scarified, of a leaf-paste made with cold water from the leaves of *Paarde praam*, or from those of *Clematis*; and the lichen *ubu-Lembu belitye* is also employed externally.

Internally, a decoction of the roots *Paarde praam* is used along with its leaf-paste.

MEDICATED BATHS.

Hot baths, medicated with a decoction or a hot infusion of certain plant substances, or simply with the plants themselves, and fomentations with the same, form a peculiarity in the mode of treatment adopted by certain Kaffir specialists. It is now known that drugs introduced directly into the blood act with a rapidity and a certainty which contrasts with the attempt to introduce them through the stomach. The number of substances employed in hypodermic injection is proof of a change in medical opinion on this point. The extreme absorbent power of the skin is also recognized. Taking both these things into account, it might be of service to employ medicated baths and fomentations in the treatment of certain maladies.

(See SCROFULA and COLDS.) The following plants are called *um-Hlambezo* as being used for fomentation.

STITCH.

Dianthus, The pink.   *Agapanthus*.

There are several species of the native Pink, which will serve the purpose, the roots usually large; and more than one variety of *Agapanthus*. The roots of both mixed are pounded and beaten up in *cold* water till they froth, and this is applied as a fomentation for severe pain in the bowels, or for stitch; and also over the body for loss of power arising from some sort of paralysis. A mere trace of the liquid is at the same time given internally.

STITCH.

Sebœa crassulaefolia—Kaffir, *ili-Bulawa*.
(See SNAKE-BITE.)

Lithospermum—Kaffir, an *i-Yeza lihlaba*.

This is a small plant with narrow linear leaves 6—8 lines long, hardly a line wide, very rough and bristly, stems pubescent.

These plants are used for stitch, *i-hlaba*, an infusion in each case.

A RASH.

Matricaria nigellaefolia, D C.—Kaffir, *um-Hlonyane womlambo* (river worm-wood), or *um-Solo womlambo*.

(See MILT-ZIEKTE.) This plant is used as a remedy for a sort of rash called in Kaffir *uku-Dliwa ngumlambo*, Bite-of-the-river. In respect of this use the plant is frequently called *um-Solo*, although this term is applied to some other plants. Why the rash in question is called by such a name is not apparent, unless it is supposed to be occasioned by a chill.

Samolus Valerandi, Lin.—*Worldwise*.

The corolla of this small plant is salver-shaped, white, the limb 5-cleft, with alternating scales.

The plant is found at Toleni and elsewhere, and is used as a remedy for the same rash.

BONE FRACTURE.

Plumbago—Kaffir, *um-Ti wamadoda*.

The common *Plumbago* shrub with its gay light-blue flowers is well known. The roots roasted like coffee are employed in inoculating the skin above a fracture of the bone, no doubt a mere counter-irritant to prevent inflammation. The same sort of inoculation is also practised occasionally in stitch. Certain experts profess to know a really important remedy for bone-fracture, but it has not been ascertained what plant they employ.

SLOW ABSORPTION.

Some medicines such as phosphorus, iron, and those plant substances which serve as blood purifiers, are admitted into the blood in small quantity and are subsequently assimilated very slowly. The principle of administering them in such a manner as to admit of slow absorption has not been acted on as it ought to be. If a considerable dose of these medicines is given, in greater part it is at once thrown out in the secretions, after doing local mischief somewhere. The doses administered ought to be very small, and the period over which this is continued should count by weeks rather than by days. Plant remedies according to native use are frequently successful in removing malignant sores and eruptions, but occasionally after a time something else makes its appearance, such as caries of the bone, which is thought to be another thing altogether, but is really the same malady in a different form. In such cases the plant antidote if necessarily given in strong doses at first, should have been continued afterwards for some length of time in very small doses, until the dregs of the poison in the blood had been destroyed.

ATROPA BELLADONNA.

Atropa Belladonna—Deadly Nightshade.

This is not a South African plant, but is referred to because some light may be thrown on one of its uses from the properties and use of several of the Solanums, employed medicinally in this country.

Hahnemann turned this plant to some account in propping up his homœopathic theory. He observed that belladonna produced in healthy persons a red rash resembling that of scarlet fever, with which he identified it. He also found that persons dosed with belladonna during a scarlet fever epidemic escaped an attack. There is, however, a weak link in his chain of proof. The rash is not identical in these two cases, and there are other sorts of red rash different from both, such as that produced in some persons by eating bitter almonds, ascribed to prussic acid.

Still, throwing his theory out of count, belladonna may be of importance in scarlet fever after all, and since it is in fact used, an analogous employment of some other Solanums may give a better direction to its use.

Solanum Melongena, S. Sodomaeum, S. Capense, S. nigrum, and perhaps others are employed as bacteria killers, or as destructive of low forms of animal life. Judging from this, may not belladonna have a special aptitude to kill the streptococcus or chain-micrococcus, believed to be the cause of scarlet fever? If so, in place of being used in the haphazard way of "doing good" in this fever, it would be used with an intelligible object and naturally in a different manner, and belladonna might well be used as a prophylactic by nipping the poison germ in the bud, for when the malady is epidemic many persons show by some symptom or other, that the infection in some shape flies about.

CHAPTER XXIII.

[CHAPTER XX—XXIII ARE ON PLANTS USED AS ANIMAL MEDICINES.]

LUNG-SICKNESS.

Phytolacca stricta—Kaffir, *um-Nyanja*.

This plant is found in moist meadows. Some of the Dutch Colonists, for want of a better name, have called it the Wild Sweet-potato owing to its having large tuberous roots. This name though quite unsuitable may be quoted for the sake of popular identification. The leaves and flowers strongly resemble those of mignonette. A good distinguishing mark is the fruit, which consists when ripe of a dense cluster of transparent sessile yellow berries, near the points of the branched stem, much resembling the berries of the White Currant.

The roots have been used with marked success in curing lung-sickness. This disease can be warded off to some extent by inoculation, but it is so little curable that a serious case is regarded as nearly hopeless. One thing that shows some relation between this plant and the disease is the circumstance, that if an ox has the poison in his system, all the ordinary symptoms of lung-sickness are immediately developed, if a decoction of the roots is administered. We must not here go upon the rock on which Homœopathy, with its motto *Similia similibus curantur*, has split, by confounding the morbid symptoms of disease, with the symptoms of nature's efforts to throw it out, and we may regard the common signs of lung-sickness to be the latter.

A dose for one animal is prepared by taking 8 oz. avoirdupois of the fresh roots powdered fine, and simmering this in two quarts of water, adding from the first a spoonful of paraffin and 16 grains of powdered blue-stone (copper sulphate). An enamelled or an earthenware pot should be used, and the simmering continued till the quantity of water is reduced to one half. When this is administered the animal should be kept in the house, with forage and water beside it to come round slowly. In slight cases taken promptly this will take place very soon; bad and far gone cases may take a long time, sometimes even three weeks. If a second dose is thought necessary, it must not be given till six clear days have elapsed, else the dose repeated will kill it.

The experience of a skilful farmer with this remedy is as follows. Lung-sickness had entered his herd, and all the other remedies were employed with a fatal result in every case. This remedy was then applied in seven different cases, occurring at separate times, and although some of the cases seemed desperate, the breathing being heard at the distance of twenty paces, the animals attacked all recovered. Some years after this, on lung-sickness showing itself, he promptly got his herd, young and old, inoculated, or drenched with a small quantity of the watery serum within the pleura of a diseased animal, ready to treat any animal that might take the disease, in the manner already mentioned. More than 20 cattle were seized, and all were saved except two cows that had to be killed on account of their extreme weakness after they got over the disease. The calves did not get on so well. Ten died of the disease, 10 got over it, but were in low condition and had to be killed owing to weakness, as they had constantly to be picked up, and 10 or 12 were saved. The weak ones would probably have recovered if kept up with artificial food—milk mixed with boiled pease-meal.

A farmer in Kat River, a few miles above Blinkwater, had lung-sickness in his herd near the end of 1887, and lost 32 despite of all the remedies commonly employed, one being paraffin and milk. He then used the roots of *Phylacca stricta*, prepared as above, and brought through 18, the whole on whom the remedy was tried.

Lung-sickness is undoubtedly caused by poison germs present in the blood, and the difficulty lies in introducing some bacteria-killing substance into the blood to kill them. This plant appears to do so. The roots are poisonous (See MISCELLANEOUS). One farmer is known who tried this remedy with no success. He may have made a mistake in the preparation. It ought, however, to be kept in mind that when the disease has made such progress as to materially injure the lungs, no remedy can avail, however valuable it might be at an earlier stage.

CHAPTER XXIV.

GALL-SICKNESS—BLACK GALL-SICKNESS—QUARTER-ILL—RED-WATER.

GALL-SICKNESS.

Conyza ivaefolia, Less.—Kaffir, *i-Savu*—Dutch, *Oonth bosje (*Oven bush)—*The Albany gall-sick bush.*

This is a Composite with lance-shaped leaves, which are shortly stalked, pointed, tapering to the base, serrate, teeth callous at the tip, smooth, 2—3 inches long. The plant is resinous and rather woody. The heads are numerous, small, and have a white effect, until they are fully opened, owing to the scales of the involucre, flowers afterwards yellowish. The Dutch name is from the stalks being employed to sweep out an oven.

A decoction is used for gall-sickness, about six tops, to which is added a small quantity of *Padde klauw* (See SNAKE-BITE) and of *Chenopodium ambrosioides* (See MISCELLANEOUS). *Teucrium Africanum*—Dutch, *Padde klauw.*

Farmers use a decoction of this plant for gall-sickness in calves, and also in sheep. A number of sheep it is said had fallen in with a quantity of this plant, and strangely their eating it produced gall-sickness. They were cured with a decoction of the root, after taking which no more died. This allegation can be taken at what it is worth. At least the whole plant should be employed in gall-sickness.

Scilla lancedefolia—Kaffir, *in-Qwebebana.*

This is a bulbous plant belonging to the Liliaceæ. The leaves are rather broad at the base, but taper, are close to the ground, and spotted over with black spots. The flower stalk is 5 or 6 inches high, with a spiked raceme of purplish flowers.

A decoction of the leaves, not the bulb, is used for gall-sickness.

Sideroxylon inerme, Lin.—*White Milk-wood*—Dutch, *Wit Melk-hout*—Kaffir, *um-Qwashu.*

This tree is common in the Eastern forests. It has small, white, axillary flowers, calix 5-parted, corolla 5-cleft; fruit a berry. The leaves are oblong, blunt, leathery, and smooth.

A decoction of the bark is used for gall-sickness.

Leonotis ovata—Dutch, *Klip dagga* (See SNAKE BITE.)
Cluytia hirsuta—Kaffir, *ubu-Hlungubedila* (See MILT-ZIEKTE.)

An infusion of the leaves of these two plants mixed is used for gall-sickness.

In-Nyongwane and *ubu-Hlungu bedila.*

The root of the former (See STOMACH), and the leaves of the other (See MILT-ZIEKTE) mixed, are used for gall-sickness.

Capparis citrifolia—a Caper-bush—Kaffir, *in-Tsihlo*.

This is a large shrub or small tree found in the Eastern Districts, occurring near King William's Town and near Main. The twigs are velvety, with ovate leaves, 1—1½ inches long, downy above, more so beneath, having for stipules two sharp hooks. The berry is larger than that of the wait-a-bit thorn. The shrub is a humble relative of the caper-bush, the berries of which were used to stimulate appetite.

A decoction of the roots is used as a remedy for gall-sickness.

Pittosporum viridiflorum, Sims—Kaffir, *um-Kwenkwe*.

This tree is plentiful in the thickets of Katberg and of Chumie Peak. The leaves, usual size 2¼ inches by ⅞ inch, are obovate, some of them pointed, some rounded, tapering towards the stalk, leathery, dark green and glossy above, the margin sometimes revolute. Flowers yellow-green; fruit, 5—6 lines long, bright orange, with 2—6 hard angular red seeds immersed in a transparent sticky resinous substance.

A decoction of the bark is an antidote for black gall-sickness.

Polygonum tomentosum, var. *glabrum*.

The genus *Polygonum* is allied to *Rumex*, and this plant will be easily recognized from its having the leaves and general characters of the *Dock*, but is quite erect, 3—4 feet high, with a red stem. It is found near streams and in moist places near Lovedale and in Tembuland.

A decoction of the entire plant is employed for black gall-sickness.

Withania somnifera, Dun.—Kaffir, *ubu-Vumba*—Fingo, *u-Vimba.*

(See SORES.) A decoction of the roots is used for black gall-sickness. As in most plants, the virtue lies in the bark of the roots, not in the stringy portion.

QUARTER-ILL.

Noltea Africana, Reich.—Kaffir, *i-Palode* (i-palo elide,) or *i-Yeza lesi-Diya.*

This tree is found in various parts of the Colony. It is plentiful in the Nqayi valley near Lovedale, and on the banks of the Chumie and of the Balfour river, as well as on the Katberg. Its natural situation is near a stream. In general appearance it somewhat resembles the wild cherry, with dark green leaves paler beneath. The leaves are oblong, elliptical, serrate; the smaller branches are purplish on the side exposed to sun light. The small white flowers have five petals, five stamens, and a five cleft calyx. The fruit is a drupe the size of a large pea, 3-lobed, with the lobes keeled.

I-Palode is an antidote for the disease called "quarter ill," or spons-ziekte. The preparation is a decoction of the leaves, of which half a quart bottle is administered when cool. This is both employed as a remedy for the disease, and as a prophylactic to ward off the malady from cattle exposed to infection. The Kaffirs think that it would be enough to scatter the branches about the kraal, probably assuming that the cattle would eat them. Some persons use the roots and not the leaves. This remedy is worthy of the attention of European farmers. It has been kept secret, and considerable sums of money have been given for the application of the remedy, where the plant used has not been disclosed.

RED-WATER.

Buphane toxicaria, Herb.—Kaffir, *in-Cwadi*—Dutch, *Gift-bol.*

(See MISCELLANEOUS.) The disease named Red-Water, in Kaffir *um-Bendeni,* and *amanzi abomvu,* has been treated with this bulb by itself. No plant remedy, however, has been so effective to prevent this disease, or cure it, as administering 40 drops of crystallized Carbolic acid thoroughly blended with one ℔. of raw Linseed oil, and also using 1 ℔. of Epsom salts in 3 bottles of warm water; one to mix with the acid and oil, and two to wash down with. Everything depends on prompt treatment.

Acocanthera Thunbergii or *Toxicophloea Thun.*—*Bushman's Poison-bush*—Kaffir, *in-Tlungunyembe.*

(See SNAKE-BITE.) A Dutch farmer, Mr. Nortje, employed the leaves of the Poison-bush and the bark of a tree named *Zeep-bast, um-Kwenkwe,* in the cure of oxen attacked with

Red-Water. The dose was a decoction of a small handful of the leaves and a strip of the bark. A pinch of gunpowder was also given to be washed down with the decoction. The sulphur in it would be useful and the saltpetre is diuretic. He succeeded with forty cases running. He was probably not aware, that much of the poisonous glucoside, the active principle in Acocanthera, had been reduced to glucose by boiling else he had not been so liberal in the quantity of leaves he employed.

CHAPTER XXV.

SCANTY MILK—CALVES—DISTEMPER.

SCANTY MILK.

Sarcostemma viminale, E. Mey.—Kaffir, *um-Belebele.*

This Asclepiad is found climbing among the branches of trees. It is not uncommon in the scrub near Lovedale, and below Katberg. Its stems are round, long, branched, as thick as a lead-pencil, leafless, and full of milky juice. The corolla is yellowish, 5-parted, the seed-vessels are 5—6 inches long, tapering, fixed in pairs on the stem at a very obtuse angle.

This plant is put to a very singular use. When a cow gives scanty milk or none at all, a number of soft stems are broken and bruised in cold water, which is administered.

It is stated that the same is done with persons. The name *um-belebele* is derived from *i-bele*, a breast or teat. It is open to doubt, whether the property mentioned gave rise to the name, or whether the name taken from the milky juice occasioned a belief in the property.

CALVES.

Myaris inaequalis. Presl.—Kaffir, *um-Nukambiba*—Dutch, *Limoen hout.*

(See MISCELLANEOUS.) The wealth of the Kaffirs lay in cattle, and their ideas on the management are founded on observation, and are worthy of attention. They took note that the calves of fatherland cows frequently die, and they ascribed this to the cows producing so much milk, that the calves got too much, and the milk turned into clots. To expel these, they take the bark of the root of *um-Pafa* (*Zizyphus mucronata*, the *wait-a-bit thorn*) and after scraping off the rind make it into a paste. They also make a paste of the leaves of *um-Nukambiba*. Of these two pastes mixed they make a hot infusion, and administer in one day a quart bottle of this, dividing it into four doses.

Solanum Capense, Thunb.—Kaffir, *um-Tumana.*

This is a low trailing bush not exceeding a foot in height, with spreading branches frequently lying on the ground. It is very prickly. The leaves are lobed, about 1¼ inch long by ½ inch wide. The flowers are small and white. It bears a light red naked berry the size of a large pea. The berry when unripe has the end next the stalk white, the other end green; thus reversing the arrangement found in some other species.

The juice of the berry is used for distemper in dogs. A paste of the leaves is also applied for sore eyes in dogs, and for old sores in people.

I-Tshongwana, a small species of *Xysmalobium* is also employed in Distemper. A decoction of the root is used, and is followed almost immediately by vomiting.

CHAPTER XXVI.

BOTS IN HORSES—GLANDERS—SORES—WORMS.

BOTS.

Gunnera perpensa, Lin.—Kaffir, *i-Puzi lomlambo*, or River pumpkin.

Clematis brachiata, Thunb. — *Traveller's joy* — Kaffir, *i-Tyolo*.

The first of these plants is found in swampy places and in ditches. Its leaves are stalked, kidney-shaped, resembling those of a species of pumpkin—whence its Kaffir name—varying according to moistness of situation from 4 to 12 inches in breadth. It bears numerous spikelets of small flowers arranged on a common flower stalk. The roots are *yellow*, fleshy, ⅔ to 1 inch in diameter, and in considerable quantity where the soil is constantly

M

wet and spongy. They dry up very rapidly, when taken out and exposed to the air.

Clematis is a well known climber with cream-coloured blossoms. The species *brachiata* is common in the Eastern Districts. It is found near streams or in moist situations, and its blossoms load the air with an agreeable fragrance. The feathery tails of its carpels make it conspicuous in autumn.

These two plants are used together for expelling bots from horses. The bot-fly, *Œstrus equi*, toward the end of summer deposits its eggs on the hair covering the knees, the inside of the fore legs, and the chest of the horse, which in biting and licking these parts introduces them into its mouth. The small worms, produced from the eggs, hook themselves to the inner coat of the stomach, and are developed into what are called bots. At the end of the following spring the bots lose their hold and pass down, and after going through the usual transformations become flies, again to go the same round.

There are veterinary surgeons who say it is impossible to expel these parasites before they quit their hold at the natural time; that unless in excessive quantity they do a horse little harm; and that when bots are supposed to cause death, the real cause is some other disease. Farmers maintain the exact contrary of these opinions, and they have truth on their side so long as they hold to observed facts, but go wrong when they make inferences from them. They suppose that a certain naturally bare place in the stomach of a horse is made so by bots, and that they kill by piercing the stomach. These conclusions are both erroneous, for bots have no means of doing either of those things. The opinions of veterinary surgeons, however, are more inexcusably wrong, as coming from professional men. It certainly does some harm when bots feed on the nutriment which ought to go to support the horse, but these parasites cannot be where they are—hooked on to the stomach—without irritating the glands and interfering with the secretion of the gastric juice, so that the horse falls off in condition. They must also poison the horse to some extent, either from exuding, as most insects do, a noxious saliva which prepares their food, or by their fæces, and the horrid smell they give out when the stomach of a horse infested with them is opened is suggestive of poisoning. The unhealthy appearance of a horse so infested is a proof of poisoning, and the parallel case of tape-worm being always accompanied with malaise suggests that with bots it is similar.

That bots may cause death, the case mentioned below under Hemp affords proof, for the horse in question was in a moribund state, turning up the white of his eyes, and yet he became well presently on their expulsion. Horses are also known to have been lean and haggard, as well as obviously suffering, from being infested with bots, and when they were expelled to have become well and strong.

When a horse shows signs of being infested by bots, a decoction to expel them may be made from two to three ounces of the fresh tubers of *i-Puzi lomlambo*, to which is added an infusion of the shoots and leaves of *Clematis*, a small handful of which must be broken up and bruised in *cold* water. This is a sufficient dose for one animal. It is better to have fresh tubers, though that is not essential; but of the dry roots less must be used. The action of this medicine is similar to that of the Male fern in expelling tape worm. The bots are dislodged either sickened or dead. It requires a rather nice adjustment to poison the bots without poisoning the horse. Still, this may be done safely, unless the root of a wrong plant is taken. Tartar emetic will expel bots. This however is a dangerous remedy, as a slight overdose will kill a horse.

The bark of *um-Kwenkwe* (See GALL-SICKNESS) is sometimes used for *i-Puzi lomlambo*, along with *i-Tyolo*, but is neither so good nor so safe.

Cannabis sativa—Hemp or Common *Dagga*—Kaffir, *um-Ya*.

The Hemp plant is found in gardens or in waste ground outside. It has dark green leaves and greenish flowers, and should not be confounded with Wild or Rooi Dagga (Leonotis) with its whorls of red flowers, though the leaves of both are smoked, and both are called *dagga*.

To expel bots, one pound of the darkest brown sugar is put into a quart of new milk (boiled milk will not do), and this is administered to a horse. A decoction made from one handful of *um-Ya*, hemp leaves, is given an hour afterwards. As the horse may become intoxicated and fall, he is placed among straw where he cannot receive any injury. The action of this remedy is much more rapid than the former which however has proved effective in many instances.

A very different use has been found for the Hemp plant.

Arsenic is employed in Styria for giving horses a glossy coat. A substitute safer and quite as good has been discovered here in hemp leaves. They are cut fine and sprinkled over the forage. The effect is to keep horses in excellent condition, and give them a glossy appearance. Besides this, it can be used to remove the winter coat of long hair, if horses are stabled and do not require to be exposed. It is presumed that in using hemp, the horses are properly fed and well treated. The leaves have the same stimulating effect as hemp-seed has when given to singing birds.

Amygdalis Persica—The Peach.

Peach leaves form perhaps the most effectual, and the safest cure for bots. Their virtue lies in the prussic acid they contain. A strong decoction is made with two double handfuls in as much water as by boiling in will fill two bottles. The whole is administered early in the morning, and half a bottle of raw linseed oil is given as a laxative an hour afterwards. This remedy has been employed successfully with the horses of the Cape Mounted Police.

GLANDERS.

Cluytia. Ranunculus.

There is a shrub of the genus *Cluytia*, found at the edge of the Hog's Back forests, which has proved effective in the hands of a Basuto in curing several known cases of glanders. Its leaves are not larger than those of *C. Hirsuta*, ovate; the seed capsule is much larger, $\frac{1}{3}$ inch in diameter, and rougher with tubercles. The root is yellow with a red bark, and is much more scorching in its properties than any of the Lasiosiphons, and gives out a pungent odour, especially when breathed on. The whole plant has an odour. The specimens brought were too imperfect to determine the species.

The dose for glanders is a small handful of the powdered roots, given internally in a decoction of a small quantity of *Ranunculus* leaves.

There are various other plant remedies for glanders, such as *um-Kwenkwe* bark, or *um-Tumana* roots, or *Klip dagga* leaves, each with *ityolo* (Clematis), and other combinations more elaborate; but that they are of any real value is very doubtful. As some veterinary surgeons of repute pronounce shooting to be the best cure for this malady, it may not be out of place to quote a native use of European appliances. A Fingo well skilled in the management of horses employed the following with success:—A table-spoonful of Stockholm tar, with a tea-spoonful of balsam of sulphur, is administered in milk. This is repeated three times, or oftener, at intervals of a day. Balsam of sulphur is sold by chemists; but it is Flowers of sulphur, 1 part; Olive oil, 4 parts; boiled to the consistence of a thick balsam.

SORES.

Withania somnifera, Dun.—Kaffir, *ubu-Vumba*—Fingo, *u-Vimba*.

This is a plant found in gardens and near houses, 3 feet high, with ovate leaves. It may readily be recognized from its bright red berries, which are enclosed like the Cape gooseberry in the inflated calyx, through which the red berries can be seen when ripe, as it is then translucent. The plant has a decided virtue in curing the sores on the backs of horses produced by being chafed with the saddle. It has been employed with effect in numerous cases. The mode of preparing it is to take the green berries, leaves, and small twigs, moisten and pound them to a paste. This is applied to the sore, and will act better if covered up and kept moist. It may take time according to the character of the wound. When the scab is formed, a simple salve will be helpful. The plant is sedative, and perhaps antiseptic.

Hypoxis sericea, and *H. obliqua*—Kaffir, (both) *i-Xalanxa*.

(See MISCELLANEOUS.) The small bulbs of *H. sericea* are roasted on the fire till an oil oozes out. This is used for anointing wounds on horses when the skin is chafed, and is highly spoken of. The large bulbs of *H. obliqua* are hollowed out, and water is put in. These are placed by the fire till the water boils, which is used for washing bad wounds.

A decoction of Blue-gum leaves has proved effective in healing severe wounds in horses as when they come down on their knees, and it must be well rubbed in. That is due partly to its being antiseptic.

A leaf-paste of an *i-Dwara*—*Senecio latifolius*, (See WOUNDS) is used for sore backs in horses.

WORMS.

Heteromorpha arborescens, Cham. and Schlecht.—Kaffir, *um-Bangandlela*.

(See SCROFULA.) A decoction of the inner bark, or of the bark of the roots, is employed to expel thread worms in horses. It is looked upon as valuable for the purpose.

Emex spinosa, Campd.—Kaffir, *in-Kunzane*.

(See STOMACH.) To expel thread worms in horses, a good handful of the leaves is put into two quarts of water and boiled down to one. A pint is sufficient for one dose. It is strong.

AN ASTRINGENT.

Pelargonium reniforme—Dutch, *Rabassam*, vulg. *Rabas*.

(See DYSENTERY.) The root of this Pelargonium wrapped in muslin and tied with twine along the bit will put a stop to purging in horses on a journey. Its juice mingles with the saliva and is swallowed. The station for this species is a soil of crumbling rock. Another species found in moist localities, *Pelargonium pulverulentum* (MISCELLANEOUS) will serve the same purpose.

A Dutch remedy for the purging of horses on a journey is to throw a small quantity of ground coffee into the horse's mouth, and repeat this two or three times after intervals.

CHAPTER XXVII.

[MISCELLANEOUS.]

FIRE STICKS—MLANJENI'S CHARMS—LIGHTNING SHRUB—
ASSEGAI WOOD—ANTI-BUG PLANT—CONVOLVULUS—FAMINE
ROOT—FIXING ON ASSEGAI HEADS—MISTLETOE—WITCH-
DOCTORS' PLANTS — THREAD — A SUPERSTITION—PLANT
POISONOUS TO CATTLE—PLANTS SAID TO BE EATEN BY VUL-
TURES—SCENTED PLANTS—FOR ECONOMIC USES.

FIRE-STICKS.

Brachylaena elliptica, Less.—Kaffir, *isi-Duli*.
Ficus Capensis, Thunb.—Kaffir, *u-Luzi*.

These were the most commonly used fire-sticks. *Isi-Duli* is a tree, the leaves of which are dark green and glossy above, woolly and white beneath, and intensely bitter. The leaves are oblong, wedge-shaped at the base, with three short lobes at the apex, sinuate and toothed at the margin; but they vary extremely in size and form. *U-Luzi* belongs to the Fig family, and its small fruits show their fig character in section.

These fire-sticks yield a kind of dust, when a pointed stick is moved rapidly forwards and backwards in a groove. The dust turns brown, then red-hot, and can be blown with tinder into a flame. This process of fire-making is called *u-Zwati*. The method of making the upper stick revolve rapidly with pressure may also have been employed. Both the process and the kinds of wood used will likely soon be forgotten.

MLANJENI'S CHARMS.

Pelargonium pulverulentum, Colv.—Kaffir, *i-Kubalo lika-Mlanjeni*.

The leaves of this Pelargonium are broadly ovate, cordate at the base, lobed, crenate, ribs very prominent on the back of the leaf, velvety above with extremely short hairs, pubescent with soft hairs beneath. They are thickish and soft, with a narrow red border more visible above. The root is fleshy, in section of a purplish colour with a white ring. The plant is common in Kaffraria, and is found on the Katberg.

This plant has a certain historic interest in connection with the Kaffir war of 1850. The prophet Mlanjeni persuaded the Kaffirs, that the roots of this plant by simply pointing them towards the English would ward off their bullets, and wet the charge in their guns so that they would not go off. The Kaffirs also tied a root round their necks so as to hang just below the throat, and they sometimes chewed the roots; with the same object in view. Possibly Mlanjeni's attention had been called to this plant when a boy, as the Kaffir herd-boys chew the leaves, which have an agreeable acid taste. *I-Kubalo* means a charm. Mlanjeni also prepared with his incantations and gave out many pieces of the Plumbago—*umti wamadoda*—for the same purpose. Some of the Kaffirs were found chewing these pieces while being shot.

LIGHTNING-SHRUB.

Cluytia pulchella, Müll.—*Lightning-shrub*—Kaffir, um-Fiyo.

This Cluytia is a shrub growing to the height of 4—5 feet. The flowers are very small, with five whitish petals, and a calyx of 5 semi-transparent imbricated sepals. A characteristic mark of *Cluytia* is the 2—3-fid glands between the petals, seen with a botanical glass. The fruit is the size of a peppercorn. This species has the leaves less distinctly reticulated than the others of the same genus, nearly round, $1\frac{1}{8}$ inch long by 1 inch wide but often much less, soft, smooth, and seen with transmitted light to be dotted all over. The bark of the young twigs is green.

To ward off lightning from striking a hut or a kraal, the Kaffirs burn the roots in the fire, and hang up branches of the shrub round the eaves of the hut, and on the kraal fence. This is done at the instance of the witch-doctors. The plant does not seem to be used in medicine. When the roots are put on the fire, they give out an excessively pungent odour, and that may have originated the notions about the plant.

ASSEGAI-WOOD.

Grewia occidentalis—*Assegai-wood*—Dutch, *Kruisbesje*—Kaffir, *um-Nqabaza*.
Ehretia Zeyheriana—Kaffir, *um-Hleli*.

Um-Nqabaza is easily recognized by its fruit which consists of one fleshy covering drawn over four seeds. The berries are yellow and sweet when ripe, and are eaten. The arrangement of the four stones in the berry gives rise to the name *kruisbesje*. The leaves are ovate pointed, crenate. The flowers are purple, with a central column of numerous stamens, conspicuous from the yellow anthers. The wood of this tree was used by the Kaffirs in making handles to their assegais. The properties for which it is selected are that it is light, flexible, easy to cut when fresh, and tough afterwards. *Curtisia faginea*, Ait. is the so called assegai-wood, but in whatever way it came to bear this name, it is denied, so far at least as the Gaika Kaffirs are concerned, that it has any connection with assegais, and it is not well fitted to make the handles from being heavy and inflexible. It should not be supposed, however, that the Kaffirs never used any wood for assegai-handles except *um-Nqabaza*, which might not always be obtainable.

Um-Hleli, a shrub or small tree, is very conspicuous from its clusters of lilac flowers light-coloured within and much darker on the outside. These are followed by bunches of green berries, blackish on one side, which turn bright-red when ripe. The corolla is salver-shaped with a long tube.

The wood was highly valued for making assegai-handles, even more so than that of the former. It is tough and flexible.

ANTI-BUG PLANT.

Chenopodium ambrosioides, Lin.—*Goose-foot*—Fingo, *um-Hlahlampetu*—Kaffir generic name for the Chenopodiums, *im-Bikicane*.

There are two types of this plant, which are very different though they have not been ranked as distinct species. One of them, apparently not the one now referred to, is noticed by Pappe. *Um-Hlahlampetu* is found in maize and Kaffir-corn fields, has the leaves oblong and fingered at the sides, the stem often red, branched, standing singly, and has an extremely pungent aromatic odour, quite different from that of the other, as well as much stronger. The other is found by waysides and in ditches, forms a bush, and has ovate, pointed, deeply serrate leaves which have a nauseous smell. This sort is used as an ingredient in animal medicines.

Um-Hlahlampetu has properties similar to those of *Pyrethrum rosaceum Caucasicum*, the tops of which ground to a fine powder form Insect Powder—that sold by Keating is best known—which destroys bugs and other insect pests. The virtue of Insect Powder has been exaggerated on the one hand, and its efficacy doubted on the other. It certainly kills flies if sprinkled on the cross-bars of a window frame, and it sickens and drives away fleas and other pests, but it is doubtful if it can kill them. If rubbed on so as to make a narrow stripe round the feet of an iron bedstead, it forms a barrier which no creeping pest will cross. Those Kaffirs to whom this property of *um-Hlahlampetu* is known, use the entire plant fresh. The proper way is to strip off the seeds and their integuments from the tops, when they ripen and turn yellow, and are then most pungent, but before they become dry or spoilt with frost, and pound them in a mortar or otherwise reduce them to a fine powder. The virtue lies in the aromatic oil, and were only one half of what is said of the plant by the Kaffir authorities to prove good, the plant would be of much value in this country, where it could be had quite fresh, and in any quantity, as it easily admits of cultivation. The powder should be kept in air-tight tins, or bottles.

A strong decoction of *Blue-gum* leaves along with the green seed vessels, has been found effectual in destroying bugs lodged in the seams and chinks of wood-work and of walls. It has an advantange over sulphate of iron in not injuring the wood, as it washes off.

CONVOLVULUS.

Convolvulus—The larger Convolvulus—Kaffir, *u-Boqo*.

If cows eat *u-Boqo*, their milk produces constipation. The Kaffirs for that reason prevent them from doing so.

FAMINE ROOT.

Hypoxis sericea—Kaffir, *i-Xalanxa*.

The flower of this plant is six-partite, giving it a star-like appearance, bright yellow. The leaves are radical, with parallel veins as in the other Amaryllideæ, and with a single plait. The bulb is small.

This is one of the famine roots. The bulbs are usually

roasted, but sometimes boiled. Women and children may be seen gathering them in the fields in times of famine.

When roasted an oil oozes out of the bulbs, which is applied to cure fresh wounds on the backs of horses.

FIXING ON ASSEGAI HEADS.

Pterocelastrus variabilis, Sond.—Kaffir, *i-Tywina.*

This forest tree had a use among the Kaffirs which may soon be forgotten. Among a barbarous people it was difficult to find a cement which would hold together things so unlike as wood and iron. In the arts, very elaborate compound cements are used for the purpose. In fastening the assegai head to the handle, the Kaffirs frequently used the strong tendon—*(umsundulo)* from the back of the neck of an ox to tie it on. There was another method. A hole was burnt in the shaft with the lower part of the head made red-hot. Into this was put the resin from the root of *i-Tywina* which oozes from it when it is heated. The head was then put in, and it was found to hold very firmly. The tree is recognizable by its curiously winged seeds. The leaves are very smooth, having no hairs of any sort, and hardly any veins. The upper surface of the leaf is of a darker green than the under, and the two halves of the leaf are seldom of the same size. There is a notch at the tip of the leaf.

Hypoxis obliqua—Kaffir, *i-Xalanxa.*

This is a large species with flowers of a warm yellow, and rough hairy leaves. The bulb is about 3 inches long by 1¾ inch wide, yellow in the inside, and very resinous. This resin which is got by roasting the bulbs, is employed for fastening on assegai heads. It is first allowed to become dry, and is then powdered and put into the hole made at the head of the shaft. The assegai head, on being heated and put in, remelts the resin and sticks firmly when cold. The resin from this bulb is not so good as that from the roots of *i-Tywina* (Pterocelastrus variabilis), but is easier to procure.

Viscum—Mistletoe—Kaffir, *in-Dembu.*

Curiously enough, though there are several species of the Mistletoe in Kaffir-land, out of the eleven in South Africa, the Kaffirs do not recognize in their use of the plant the distinction between the species, but pay regard to those which grow on the mimosa.

A decoction of the leaves is used for lumbago. It is said to have an effect on the secretions of the kidneys and to restore the natural colour. A decoction is also made from a twig of the species with red berries, and a tea-spoonful is taken for sore throat. A sort of bird-lime is made from the berries of the mistletoe.

The Hottentots and Malays have superstitions about this plant, and its efficacy in preparing a love philtre.

Schouw (Earth, Plants, and Man, p. 218) says of the mistletoe—"A beverage was (anciently) prepared from the mistletoe, and used as a remedy for all poisons and diseases, and which was suposed to favour fertility." There is an analogy between the beliefs in South Africa about mistletoe, and those of the Druids, almost suggestive of one origin. The Druids had regard to the mistletoe growing on the oak alone; the Kaffirs, to those on the mimosa. The beliefs about its acting as a love philtre, and other things of the same nature, are common to both. One would think that in place of the far-fetched fancies, that the mistletoe was an emblem of the new year from its green leaves showing on the bare branches, and that all the other superstitions about its virtues arose out of its use in the ancient idolatry, it was originally a medicinal plant with reputed properties which modern experience hardly confirms.

WITCH-DOCTORS' PLANTS.

Phytolacca stricta—Kaffir, *um-Nyanja*.
Cucumis Africanus, Lin.—Kaffir, *u-Tangazana*.

(For *um-Nyanja*, See LUNGSICKNESS.)

U-Tangazana is common in the fields near Lovedale, and in Kaffraria. Like other plants of the gourd family it has a long trailing branched stem, with 5-lobed leaves sometimes sub-lobed, toothed. The flowers are yellow. The pepo or gourd is small, 1½ in. by 1 in., covered with short spines 2 lines long. The whole plant is rough.

Both these are witch-doctors' plants. The preparations from them were not administered to the patient on account of any medicinal property, but simply as emetics, prior to the expulsion of the malady which the witch-doctors ascribed to the person being bewitched. The roots of *um-Nyanja* are large and tuberous—hence some of the

N

Colonists call the plant the wild sweet-potato—and a decoction of them was given in very small quantity as they are poisonous and highly dangerous. *U-Tangazana* is emetic and purgative. A decoction of the leaves was administered, dose, one-fourth of a pint; also a decoction of the root, or a few drops of the juice of the fruit, in a table spoonful of water. This also is a dangerous plant.

These plants are also animal medicines, the first of them important. The poisonous character of *um-Nyanja* is shown from a nearly fatal accident which happened at Greykirk in Kat River. Three brothers had been eating a portion of the tubers when out in the field, and were poisoned. Fortunately one of them was able to go home and report. They were recovered by giving them an emetic, though one of them was in a state of collapse. Besides the two plants just named, the Kaffir witch-doctors used another emetic, the root of a tree *Elaeodendron croceum, Saffron wood*, named *um-Bomvane* from its red roots. This was, however, for a different purpose, and was employed in trial by ordeal, *uku-Hlanjwa* or purgation. It is said that all who drank the decoction died.

They also administered a decoction of the roots of *in-Tsihlo (Capparis citrifolia)* when a person was supposed to be bewitched.

THREAD.

Gazania pinnata var. *integrifolia*—Kaffir, *um-Kwinti*— Dutch, *Boter-bloem.*

(See CHILDREN'S &c.) The long narrow leaves of this

plant have white rather tenacious fibres on each side of the midrib on the back. The Kaffirs made use of this for thread in the olden time.

Goats are fond of the leaves and flowers, and it makes them give a large quantity of rich milk.

A SUPERSTITION.

Myaris inaequalis, Presl.—Kaffir, *um-Nukambiba*—Dutch, *Limoen hout.*

This is a shrub or small tree, plentiful in Kaffraria and at Katberg. The leaves are compound, unequally pinnate. The leaflets are shortly stalked, dentate, with the two sides very unequal. With transmitted light they are seen to be dotted all over. They have a strong, not agreeable odour when bruised; contain a large amount of a volatile oil and are highly inflammable. The flowers are in panicles and are white. From a loose resemblance of the leaves some persons call this shrub bastard sneeze-wood.

The Kaffirs used to put this shrub on the fire and fumigate an infant boy with the vapour till he sneezed. They thought that would make him strong. *Um-Nukambiba* means, smell of the striped field mouse.

PLANT POISONOUS TO CATTLE.

Haplocarpha lyrata, Harv.—Dutch, *Bietouw.*

A Composite with lyrate-pinnatifid, stalked leaves, woolly and white beneath. The terminal lobe is ovate; the flowers are yellow above. The plant is found towards the Fish

River in Victoria East, in the pastures. It is regarded as poisonous to stock, and produces swelling up with flatulence. When kept down by constant grazing, no bad effects are noticed, but if allowed to grow up by the stock being removed for a time, there are likely to be deaths on their return. There seems no reason to doubt the opinion of the intelligent farmers there about this plant. Possibly the name *bietouw* may be applied elsewhere to a different plant. Its extermination seems feasible by cutting down the conspicuous flowers so as so prevent seeding, and rooting out the larger plants.

PLANTS SAID TO BE EATEN BY VULTURES.

Buphane toxicaria—Kaffir, *in-Cwadi*—Dutch, *Gift-bol*.
Senecio angulatus—Kaffir, *in-Dindilili*.

In-Cwadi is a large bulb, 6 inches high, and $3\frac{1}{2}$ broad, with a cylindrical rootstock 2 inches deep, diameter the same. It stands halfway out of the ground. The leaves are strap-shaped, tapering, 12—20 inches in length, spirally twisted, standing erect from the top of the bulb and spread out like a fan. The rootstock is said to have furnished the Bushmen with an arrow poison. The coats of the bulb are very numerous, and are thin, transparent, and silky—hence *in-Cwadi*, book. This bulb is found on the N. W. slope of Chumie Peak, on the Eland's berg, on the mountains near Main, Tembuland, and near King William's Town.

In-dindilili is a climbing plant with long stems, trailing over bushes, with fleshy, stalked, ovate leaves, wedge-shaped at the base. The flowers are yellow, in a corymb.

PLANTS SAID TO BE EATEN BY VULTURES.

Mr. W. W. Gqoba remarked to Bombo a respected sensible Kaffir of the old school, "I have often wondered how the vultures and other carrion birds can eat flesh in such a high state of putridity, and suffer no harm from it." The other replied, "They have plants which they eat for that, *in-Cwadi* and *in-Dindilili*." A Gaika Kaffir knew about this habit of vultures but did not know the plants. Another native had heard of the vultures eating *in-Cwadi*, but believed it was to sharpen their sight!

There are two questions to settle before any conclusion can be come to on a thing so novel in Natural History— Do the vultures and carrion birds eat plants at all? and, Are these the plants?

The existence of such an opinion among the Kaffirs will perhaps warrant some observations on the thing as a hypothesis. *Incwadi* is well fitted to do what is supposed. Its active principle is a germ-killer, and a powerful tonic and probably a stimulant to the action of the heart, and it would both destroy the germs in the meat, and counteract the torpefying effects of gorging by quickening the circulation and raising the temperature, which Pasteur has shown is a protection to birds against poison-germs.

In-dindilili, a Senecio, has none of these qualities. A plant substance is supposed to be a digestive to carrion birds gorged with meat, and if it is really eaten by these birds, it may serve that purpose or some other not known.

Right or wrong, the Kaffirs show penetration in these observations, and it would be worth while to look more narrowly into the habits of carrion birds.

MISCELLANEOUS.

SCENTED PLANTS.

Andropogon—Kaffir, *isi-Fikane*—Sesuto, *Somnyane*— Dutch, *Limoen gras*.
Lasiospermum radiatum, Trev.—Kaffir, An *isi-Fikane*.

One or two species of the Grass *Andropogon* are called *isi-fikane* in Kaffir. The stalks and leaves have a strong and very agreeable odour, resembling woodruff. When they are fresh, the scent from a handful will fill a room. The Kaffir women either keep this grass in the leaf form, or reduce the leaves to a powder.

The Composite *Lasiospermum* grows in drier localities than the former. It has a similar scent but much weaker. It is perennial, with leaves pinnately divided; flowers with a yellow disk and white ray.

Besides these there is a plant—flowers not seen; it may be a *Drimia*—with the dried leaves similar to the first named, and the same odour, resembling that of the Tonka bean. The bulbs are like chestnuts. It is called *Rosane*, and is found in Tembuland.

FOR MAKING SOAP, AND SKINS FOR CLOTHING.

Mesembryanthemum micranthum, Haw.—Kaffir, *i-Qina*— Dutch, *Loog*.

This is a rather low lying plant, growing in masses. The stems are partly trailing with numerous articulate branches; the leaves are nearly round in section, ¾ inch long, less than a line through, tapering to both ends, curved inwards. The calyx has 4 lobes, longer than the petals which are white. It is plentiful near Lovedale, King William's Town, and in many places. The ash is used, by the Hottentots chiefly, in making soap.

I-Qina is a generic name for various mesembryanthemums. There is a species probably *M. bellidiflorum* with 3-angled, rather awl-shaped leaves, and flowers purple in general effect, 1 inch in diameter, which is used to soften skins for clothing. They make a paste of the plant and work in the juice into the skin with a stone. The thicker part of the skin is cut or scraped off with a sharp hatchet, and the thinner remaining portion is then rubbed off with sand procured from powdered sandstone.

TENACIOUS SEWING MATERIAL.

Asparagus stipulaceus, Lam., and var., *spinescens*—an *Asparagus*—Kaffir, *im-Vane*.

This asparagus is a bush 3—4 feet high, branched, with a silvery gray bark, and straight slender spines $\frac{1}{2}$ inch long. The flowers are profuse in quantity, with an agreeable odour, small, whitish with a small green line down the middle of the six segments of the limb. Owing to the yellow anthers, collectively they look cream-coloured. The leaflets are thread-like, $\frac{1}{4}$ inch long, whorled, round, a $\frac{1}{2}$ to 1 inch long. The shrub is plentiful near King William's Town, and in Tembuland.

The roots of the Asparagus family have a tenacious core with a thick, fleshy cortical portion. The economic use of this core is to sew cracked calabashes, and for such like purposes.

This *im-Vane*, and one or two others of the same Asparagus family, have certain medicinal uses among the natives under the head of blood-purifiers. Were a preparation made from the roots, and combined with a Tonic such as Calumba, it would be of great value for the purpose of blood-purifying.

CHAPTER XXVIII.

PREPARATIONS FROM PLANTS— INFUSION—DECOCTION—TINCTURE—LEAF-PASTE — TINCTURE BY THE JOINT METHOD — PREPARATION WITH SUGAR OF MILK—POWDERS.

PREPARATIONS FROM PLANTS.

Some suggestions on the mode of making preparations from plants may be found useful.

The ordinary preparations are an Infusion, a Decoction, a Tincture, and a Leaf-paste. When a note is made here in the description of a plant, which method is to be adopted, or about anything special in the mode of preparing, that ought to be followed, though the reason may not be stated. Thus, in *Clematis*, Traveller's joy, the note is make a *cold infusion* of the leaves and leaf-stalks—not the ordinary or hot infusion, nor a decoction. The explanation is, that the pungent principle to be extracted is volatile. Hot water is therefore unsuitable, and to boil is inadmissible. When no direction is given, the thing may be regarded as uncertain, or indifferent.

INFUSION.

The parts of the plant taken for medicinal use—whether the leaves, or the bark of the stem, or of the root—should be cut down to shreds and infused exactly like tea as regards temperature and other circumstances, and just as with it care should be taken not to boil the leaves or bark, as that might expel an important volatile principle, or might extract something, such as tannin, which is not wished. In some cases a long infusion is necessary, as with orange and lemon leaves, from which a tolerable tonic preparation can be made in this way. In that case the infusion requires to be kept warm for twelve hours on or near a stove.

DECOCTION.

A decoction is made by boiling, but not quite in the usual way. So many things in nature have a relation to the boiling point of water, that decoction ought to be the keeping up of the temperature for some time to 212 deg. Fah. or 100 deg. C., or nearly so, but not very long or violent boiling, which for extracting the virtues of plants may be looked upon as excluded. At most, boiling should only be simmering. Roots especially require to be powdered, and the liquid afterwards strained. Plant substances should not be boiled in a metallic pot. Chemical action so often takes place between the metal and some substance in the plant, that an earthenware vessel or an enamelled one should always be used.

TINCTURE.

A tincture is made by steeping for a few,—some make it fourteen—days in spirits of wine. Another way is by making the alcohol percolate slowly through the plant-substance. The parts of the plant should be cut small, unless it is wished to avoid extracting too much colouring or other matter, and excepting poisonous plants, the ordinary proportion between the dry plant substance and the solvent is 1 to 8; or, a drachm to every fluid ounce. With fresh plants it is about 1 to 4; but that will depend on the weight a plant loses in drying. This will secure a uniform strength. The alcohol is usually cold. For extracting resins and essential oils, it would be better to keep it warm for a length of time. Brandy, though far inferior as a solvent to spirits of wine, is frequently employed in this country to extract the virtues of plants, as with buchu, blue-gum leaves, and some tonics. With brandy considerable heat must be applied for twelve hours in a cooking oven or near a stove. The brandy should be of the best French quality, free from harsh-tasting fusel oil, if the preparation is to be used internally.

Tinctures should be strained through muslin to remove all vegetable matter, and kept in glass-stoppered phials.

LEAF-PASTE.

To apply a paste of the leaves of a medicinal plant is rather a Kaffir peculiarity. They employ two smooth stones to make leaf-paste. A common mortar of Wedgewood ware is the most suitable thing, and a few drops of water are added, if necessary. The paste must be moist when applied, and kept by a piece of oil-cloth or other covering from drying up and thus becoming quite useless. Confusion sometimes arises from the misuse of terms. In common parlance a poultice of the leaves of a plant just means a paste of the leaves.

TINCTURE BY THE JOINT METHOD.

In some cases spirits of wine does not dissolve out properly all the ingredients in a plant. It is a good but not a universal solvent. It may be advisable with some plants first to make a tincture by steeping the parts used some days in spirits of wine, and then to make an infusion of the residue, or with more of the plant substance if it is abundant, with boiling water and allow it to stand twelve hours. This infusion should be strained and added to the tincture. There will be no difficulty about its keeping.

PREPARATION WITH SUGAR OF MILK.

It is always best when the plant can be had fresh; and there is the constant difficulty about preparations, whether they really contain every ingredient. There is good reason to believe, that if the leaves or other parts of a plant were beaten up in a mortar with sugar of milk, the composition would keep perfectly and preserve all the virtues of the fresh plant. The quantity of the plant could easily be regulated, and it would be convenient to make up the compound into tablets, each sufficient for a dose. For domestic use pure lump sugar would probably suffice. The making of sugar of milk tabloids, charged with an alkaloid, is well enough known, but except for convenience there is no advantage in this over a tincture as regards containing everything in the plant.

POWDERS.

A very common mode in South Africa of making a preparation from a plant is to reduce the leaves or root, if dry, to a powder; if fresh, to the smallest parts possible; and administer in a little water, or otherwise. Senna powder and ground ginger are familiar examples elsewhere, but here the thing is more general. There are advantages of this method. The action of the drug is more gradual, and it is preferable where the medicine is meant to mingle with the materials digested, and to enter the blood.

APPENDIX I.

CONSUMPTION AMONG CIVILIZED NATIVES.

Consumption is prevalent among civilized Kaffirs, more so apparently than among the Red Kaffirs. Its prevalence is due to a variety of causes.

1. Cases of hereditary consumption are more numerous, when a civilized community is exempted from the rigorous law of the survival of the strongest, which holds among the heathen Kaffirs.

2 Civilized natives wear European clothes, which become wet with perspiration from their working in the hot sun, and which are sometimes soaked with rain ; and they receive a mischievous chill from not shifting them.

3. Numbers of natives sleep together in the same hut, with no chimney for ventilation, and every chink closed to keep out cold. They thus breathe foul air, which produces impurity of blood from non-oxygenation. This predisposes to any prevalent form of disease.

4. The South African type of typhoid or enteric fever is accompanied by chest and liver complications. The commonness of this fever is due to infection and bad water. When the primary attack passes off, the lung complication frequently ends in consumption.

5. Other causes are the want of nourishing food, or of warm clothing and of fire in winter, and sleeping on the ground or on a mat. Persons whose nervous system is more highly developed from education cannot stand rough usage like those who lead a mere animal life. Chills and colds from some of these causes induce a form of low inflammation in the lungs, beginning behind at the bottom of the lung in many cases, which ends in the lung going into cavities.

6. Infection from consumptives in the later stages of the disease, too frequently takes hold of those who are rendered susceptible of it from the predisposing causes just mentioned.

7. There can be no doubt that giving way to vicious indulgences, drunkenness and others, brings death by consumption to many school natives. It is quite true that the

heathen Kaffirs are in these respects ten times worse; but those who are nominally Christian, and yet live like the heathen, will discover that the Christian religion kills where it does not cure.

It is evident that a rectification must take place along the whole line. The Christianized natives must have houses of several apartments, furnished with fire-places and chimneys, and educated young men must pay attention to the Laws of Health. The clothing of the natives in adopting the European dress has changed for the worse as regards health. Europeans have never discovered the unsuitability of their dress to a hot climate, because they do so little work in the hot sun and have devolved field labour on the natives. Perhaps the best thing the natives could do, would be to imitate the Syrians, Chinese, and Japanese, who wear simpler and looser under garments when actually engaged in work, and put on other articles above on ceasing from work, or as the day gets cooler. They should also at any cost of trouble shift articles of clothing which are wet with perspiration or with rain. A mistake has also been made in subjecting raw, undisciplined natives to severe brain toil in education, and it would be better for a period to accept lower attainments, than to bring upon so many an early death. For such of them as follow a sedentary occupation, or have much brain-work, a more nourishing diet and the use of tea or coffee, become a necessity.

The primary causes of consumption, which are a hereditary tendency, and infection, require more serious treatment. The most important thing here is vigilance in taking the malady in its incipient stage. One of the most important remedies at that stage is carbolic acid.

CARBOLIC ACID.

Carbolic acid is well known to be a germ-killer, but it appears to be a specific for destroying the germ which causes tubercular consumption. It is used with a Respirator. A piece of sponge is soaked in one part of carbolic acid mixed with twenty of warm water. This is placed in the respirator, and a person breathes through it. The mixture must be renewed from time to time. It is not necessary to wear the respirator constantly. The whole of the blood passes through the lungs many times in twenty-four hours, so that contact with carbolic vapour is insured to the mucous lining of the lungs, and to the blood also if there are germs in it, though the respirator is worn only part of the day. Should the vapour occasion any irritation to the lungs, two or three drops of laudanum may be put on the sponge. Creasote serves the same purpose as carbolic acid, and of it, use one drop. It appears to have a specialty in asthma.

The Respirators sold by the druggists are far too expensive for native use. An imitation sort has been made by tinsmiths in King William's Town on suggestions from the Hospital, but this also is too dear, and complex. It is of no use to make a respirator to include both mouth and nostrils—which might be necessary, were it meant to exclude cold air. A simple one for the mouth alone would be quite sufficient, as it is supposed the person who is to be benefited would choose to breathe through it, while to do so constantly, is not necessary. Many cases have been known of consumption arrested by the inhaling of carbolic acid, and it would probably be most efficacious if used on the first appearance of consumptive symptoms, where there is an inherited tendency, or there has been infection. The qualified estimate of its virtue is founded on its use in cases where it has come in far too late.

There is another very important use of carbolic acid—*to nip infection in the bud*—where a person has breathed the air of an apartment poisoned by germs from a consumptive patient.

For this, a small sponge, or piece of one, should be soaked in one part of carbolic acid to twelve of hot water, and placed in any funnel, a bottle filler would suit, or one merely of paper. The person who has undergone infection should draw five or six inspirations deep into the chest through the sponge. It is better to breathe through it both ways, as the hot breath vaporizes the carbolic acid better, and in that case the sponge retains its efficacy when dry. Once, or at most twice a day is quite enough for this experiment. Extreme caution should be used in it, as the carbolic vapour is very strong, and it might produce congestion. The inspirations may be made fewer than five or six, and the acid may be made more dilute. No pain should be produced.

Besides acting as a bacteria killer, carbolic acid has some other action. There are two gentlemen who make use of it with effect in curing obstinate colds, in neither of whom is there any trace of a consumptive tendency. It appears to reduce inflammation, and to promote the forming of mucus, in which it passes off.

The symptoms which show that the action of carbolic acid in either of the methods mentioned is beneficial, are :—

Pain in the chest is lessened.

The high pulse is reduced.

Restlessness, disinclination to settle down to do anything, and uneasy head symptoms are removed.

Acidity of breath is taken away.

There is an improved appetite.

Recent experiments have shown the value of inhaling in chest complaint a substance very different from carbolic acid or creasote—oil of peppermint. This ranks with the most powerful of the antiseptics and germ-killers. Dr. W. Leonard Braddon, in the Lancet of March 17th and 24th, 1888, reports six cases of phthisis which he had treated with inhalation of peppermint oil, 10 drops of pure oil on cotton wool, renewed every few hours, in a respirator worn in the house all day. One was cured completely in six weeks. The improvement in the other cases was encouraging. This also might be tried by the Natives. It has the advantage of being perfectly safe. The mistake of being too sanguine in expecting a cure should be avoided. Inhalation is a new departure in the treatment of consumption, but improvement may be very gradual and require patience.

A lady from England with severe chest complaint was being conveyed by her husband into the dry interior. When so far on the way, she became so ill that her

o

husband went into a Dutch farm-house, and asked whether he might bring in his wife to die. This was granted. The humane hostess, however, asked if she might treat the lady, to which her husband said, by all means if she could do anything. She accordingly swathed her in flannel moistened with raw linseed oil, and also administered some. The lady became so much better, that she turned back.

Mrs. Young of Main heard of this and used the same appliances in the case of a native girl from Gaga, near Lovedale, who was in consumption and had gone to Tembuland for a change of air, and became so ill that she was to be taken home to die. After treatment she was so much better as to go back with comfort and was since walking about at home.

Mrs. Young recommends the following treatment:— "Take a flannel cloth soaked in *raw* linseed oil, and wrap it round the trunk of the body to the chin, and put wraps over it to form a comfortable pack. At the same time administer a dessert spoonful of the oil—it must be *raw* oil, the boiled is said to be poisonous—three times a day *after food*. This should be repeated daily for some time, and the patient must keep in bed at least when in the pack. After leaving off, the oil should be rubbed into the skin very freely so that the absorption continue without check. Good diet and dry air are necessary."

It has been noted that while pulmonary disease in Europeans begins at the top of the lung, in Natives it begins at the bottom. Dr. Henry M. Chute of King William's Town, who corroborates this, states from his experience in the Port Elizabeth Hospital, that consumption in Natives often takes the form of a low inflammation, and somehow the lung goes into cavities. He is not quite sure that this malady is absolutely identical with phthisis in Europeans, though it may be closely allied to it.

The use of linseed oil in the case of Native consumptives is worthy of a trial. Should it succeed, it may prove to be the revival of an old remedy. Anointing with oil as practised in the ancient Church may after all be more than a ceremony, and it should not be supposed that *any* oil would serve.

APPENDIX II.

ON SOME PECULIARITIES OF THE AFRICAN RACE.

In the basins of the Congo and of the Zambesi, in Sierra Leone, the white man's grave, and in other fever-haunted tracts of tropical Africa, the African enjoys an exemption from malaria fever, as compared with other races of men, or takes it in a milder form. But for this fatal scourge invaders would have come in and trampled down and destroyed the native tribes, so that we may look on malaria fever as the salvation of the African race. It cannot be from any superior strength of lungs, or spleen or other of the vital organs, for in these they are no stronger than other men. In one point, however, the African stands alone. He has a very thick, fully developed skin—not the cuticle so much as the *rete mucosum* layer and the true skin

—a far more effective organ for all the functions of the skin, than other men possess.

The importance of the skin in relation to malaria fever is shown from the following fact. When travellers are crossing a hot malarious plain, it is not uncommon for them to pass through without an attack of fever; but after they reach the pure air of the hills to have an attack then, frequently fatal. The cause of this is, that while they are in the plain breathing the hot air, they are bathed in perspiration from morning to night, and they exhale the poison through the pores of the skin. When they reach the cool bracing air of the hills, the skin becomes dry, the malaria poison imbibed before accumulates in their veins, and they have an attack. What they ought to do is to keep up for a period the perspiration by swathing themselves with folds of flannel, and they should continue taking quinine long after they have ceased to breathe malarious air.

The function of the skin in eliminating poisons from the blood is well known, but the above shows its special importance in relation to the germs of malaria fever. The African possesses an abnormally thick skin, which from being a larger and more developed organ does its work much more effectually, and hence his system can throw out the malaria poison.

It is a mistake to suppose that the power of the African to resist malaria is the mere result of habit. No doubt habit is one element, but South African natives from tracts where malaria fever is unknown, stand a malarious climate better than white men.

Another peculiarity of the African is the blackness of his skin. Black is the coolest colour. If several closed tin vessels painted with various colours, one left of bright tin, have been filled with boiling water, the black one will cool soonest by radiation, a white one, or one of bright tin, will retain the heat longest, as being the worst radiator. Black is both the best radiator and the best absorbent; white the worst in both.

Nature is peculiarly careful in keeping the temperature of the blood down at 98 deg. Fah.; 102 deg. produces inflammatory action, and 105 deg. is fever heat, with development of bacteria. Were the chief danger from the heat of the sun, black would not be a good colour for the skin, as it is the best absorbent; but the sun's heat can be warded off by white clothing, by pith helmets, and by turbans. The chief sources of heat, which cannot be got rid of, are the vital heat, and the breathing of hot air. Black is the best colour for a hot climate as being the best radiator of heat, and it is a colour-aid to the action of the skin in keeping down the temperature of the body by perspiration sensible and insensible, in which functions the skin of the African is a more effective organ than that of other races. The way in which Africans cower over a fire in cold weather is an additional proof that black is a cool colour.

APPENDIX III.

FRUITS IN RELATION TO CLIMATE.

There is a notable relation between fruits and the climate in which their growth is natural, such that they serve important purposes there, and are of little use elsewhere.

THE MANGO.

The mango is grown in India, and belongs to the equatorial belt. On first eating the mango, one may notice it has a pronounced taste of turpentine. This property stands in immediate relation to a hot climate. When the temperature of the air is 85 deg. F. or more, if a person goes about much the skin is constantly clammy with perspiration which is weakening, or else if he is still, fluid accumulates in the body so much, that indentations made in the skin remain for sometime—a sort of skin dropsy. Were diuretics used to get rid of superabundant fluid, the excessive stimulation would be followed by a reaction, and the constitution would soon be injured. For this Nature provides a remedy in the form of a fruit, to which a diuretic is added in small quantity, so that it does its work and is followed by no injury. That turpentine, tar, and some of the resins are diuretic is well known. It may be objected, that by culture the finer kinds of the mango lose this turpentine flavour. This, however, is merely a comparative thing, the quantity only being reduced, which allows of a greater amount of the fruit being eaten.

THE ORANGE.

The mango is named here for the sake of pointing out the principle that fruits have relation to the wants of man in the climate in which they grow; and the orange, though naturalized, is a South African fruit. Its range is from the latitude of Spain, on the one side, and from that of South Africa on the other, to the Equator. The fruit of the same family—the lime, the lemon, the citron, and the shaddock—occupy a similar area, only that the lime as being more tender to frost is found in the hotter portion, and the lemon which is hardier in the cooler. All these have the same acids, chiefly citric, but the orange has more sugar. The orange family form practically the only Winter fruits, though some have fancied that summer was rather the season for a cool acid drink. The orange has several very different properties. It supplies an acid (citric) just when the cold winds set in and stop perspiration and the activity of the skin, and put a greater strain on the liver, while at the same time vegetables become scarce. Combined with this there is a tonic, stimulant, volatile oil, and a bitter natural principle, hesperidin, contained chiefly in the outer rind. The tonics prepared from this are well known under the names of Tinctura and Syrupus Aurantii. The " orange cure " is known in South Africa, but not so well as it ought to be. Persons using the orange medicinally take about eight a day, and these not too sweet. They exhilarate as much as brandy would, and one would fancy are rather more wholesome. There are some who are well only from the beginning to the end of the orange season. They might maintain health during the interval by the use of lime juice and hot-water with sugar in dyspepsia, or without sugar if there is inactivity or disorder of the liver. A tonic of great value is made by boiling six lemons, cut in halves, for an hour in a quart of water, with sugar according to taste. Marmalade retains the tonic virtue of the fruit from which it is made.

THE PEACH.

The peach, also naturalized in South Africa, has a narrower range. It extends from a latitude corresponding to this to as far from the equator as the south of France.

In this country peaches come to the greatest perfection in the cool upland tracts. In places where there is a hot stifling atmosphere from the middle of December to the middle of February, the peaches in ordinary seasons are utterly destroyed by maggots, as if they were not wanted in such spots. These maggots come from a clear-winged fly of the genus Tripeta, which pierces the fruit as it begins to ripen, and deposits its eggs.

The peculiarity of the peach is the presence of prussic acid in the fleshy part of the fruit. Other stone fruits contain this acid but in the kernel only. Prussic acid is a powerful sedative, and allays inflammation. Peaches dead ripe reduce inflammation in the stomach and in the bowels, and have been known to effect a complete cure in chronic dysentery. There are other effects of prussic acid used medicinally, and ripe peaches, as well as those which are dried, or preserved, may be expected to produce the same. The climate belt in which the peach grows naturally has the peculiarity of combining a hot sun with chilling winds, and a night temperature differing much from that of day. That is apt to cause irritations and inflammations, and a fruit supplying small quantities of prussic acid may have relation to this. The presence of prussic acid in the peach tree shows itself in the leaves, a decoction of which is employed to kill maggots in festering sores, and also to clean out and heal them.

THE APRICOT.

The apricot with its glossy bright green leaves is so well fitted to grow in a dry climate, that it may be looked on as the most characteristic fruit of South Africa, and admits of being produced in the greatest perfection. Of all fruits it has the most pronounced aperient properties, possessed both by the fresh fruit and also by dried apricots, boiled or stewed. A knowledge of this fact is specially useful to those who use aperients habitually. It may enable them to discontinue the use of these, or at least to have an alterative to resort to. The peculiar adaption of the apricot to the climate of this country arises from the fact that dry hot air always stimulates the liver at first, and eventually makes it more torpid. There are consequently more persons in proportion, who suffer from torpid liver and consequent constipation in this than in an English climate.

APPENDIX IV.

THE SOUTH AFRICAN HORSE-SICKNESS.

The malady known by the name of horse-sickness, like that caused by the bite of the tsetse fly, seems to be peculiar to Africa. It makes its appearance after the heat of summer, but occurs very irregularly in different years, is very fatal in autumn, but disappears with the first touch of frost. It takes the form of an acute inflammation of the lungs, and when gray looking matter comes from the nostrils the disease is speedily fatal. Horse-sickness usually runs its course very quickly after the appearance of the first symptoms, and occasionally a horse will drop down dead in harness. In these cases the malady has been going on unobserved.

Though it takes the form of an inflammation of the lungs, horse-sickness is the effect of a blood-poison and is not a mere local disease. Some of the semi-scientifics explain it by referring the malady to night chills from heavy dew and fog after hot days. This is refuted by referring to the fact, that all these secondary causes are equally prevalent in other parts of the world where horse-sickness is unknown. That it is due to a blood-poison is proved from the blood being discoloured, and from the heart and other organs, becoming soft and flabby. There are resemblances between horse-sickness and malaria fever, loose indeed but sufficient to prove an analogous origin—from a *malaria*, no doubt bacterial.

They both appear after the development of a certain degree of heat, and they disappear with an accession of cold, especially of frost.

Both are confined to certain tracts, but the nature of the spots in horse-sickness is unknown.

Both are to a good extent non-infectious.

The breezy uplands are quite exempt from both.

Exposure to night-fogs is specially likely in both to bring on an attack.

Garlic to some extent wards off both.

It is owing to its virtue in warding off malaria fever, that Spaniards and Italians living in the malarious tracts are adddicted to the use of garlic, though by tainting the blood it gives the body such a disagreeable odour. A taste for garlic has now spread more widely, but such was its origin.

We suppose then, that horse-sickness is due to a poison germ, which reproduces itself with a certain temperature. These germs are more condensed in the lower air at night, and fog probably predisposes the lungs to take them in. This will explain why stabling horses before nightfall usually saves them. The germs perhaps also fall with heavy dew on the grass, and hence it is safer not to allow horses during the sickly season to go out till the dew has risen. The blood is poisoned, but as with cholera, frequently some mishap such as excessive fatigue is required to bring on an attack. Frost kills the germs in the air and the poison soon passes out of the blood. Every zymotic disease has its special organ which it attacks—one the colon, another the spleen, but this one the lungs.

There are two ways of dealing with the disease, should it supervene despite of care in protecting horses from night fog and in preventing excessive fatigue. You may deal with the effect, or with the cause.

The effect—inflammation of the lungs—is best arrested by covering up a horse in a warm stable with blankets and bags of hot bran, and also using sudorifics, to produce a dense perspiration. If this is done in time, it is frequently effectual; but the slightest chill if allowed will be fatal. Some use blisters to stop inflammation.

The other method is to deal with the cause—the poison germs in the blood. One of the remedies used for the purpose is the following combination.

Conyza ivaefolia, Less.— Dutch, *Oonth bosje* — Kaffir, i-*Savu*.

Chenopodium ambrosioides, Lin.—Kaffir, an *im-Bikicane*.

Teucrium Africanum—Dutch, *Padde klauw*.

It is not improbable that when horse sickness is prevalent small doses of *Blepharis Capensis* or of *Crabbea cirsioides*, as well as other species of either genus, would kill the germs in the blood and ward off an attack. These plants are used by the Kaffirs in curing horse sickness. It is necessary to use caution in respect of quantity, which ought to be small. The preparation is a slight decoction of the leaves and roots. A root of garlic tied round the bit of a horse's bridle will, it is alleged, prevent this sickness, from the juice being swallowed with the saliva, and garlic leaves chopped down among forage are said to have the same effect.

APPENDIX V.

THE PASTURE AND THE GRAMINIVORA

There are some very notable differences between the pasture in England and the South African pasture. The English grasses are much richer and more juicy than those here, and they are little injured by frost and snow, but cannot stand drought. The South African grasses are dry and coarse, and the blades are rendered by frost as worthless as wood-shavings, but by means of their underlying carpet of roots they can withstand drought in a surprising manner. The meaning of this in the economy of Nature is not far to seek. The mean temperature of South Africa (60 deg.), is ten degrees above that of England (50 deg.), and were the grasses here as rich as the English grasses which require to be more nutritious to keep up the vital heat in a colder climate, the graminivora, especially the wild animals, would die of liver diseases. The nearer the equator you go, the grasses are the coarser. This principle must be taken with the qualification, that on a volcanic and on a limestone soil, the grasses are always sweeter.

The fact of such arrangement in the economy of Nature as the one mentioned, suggests that the adaptation of the pasture to the graminivora does not stop there. The pasture does not consist of mere grasses, but is studded with medicinal plants, and as these are grazed down, their medicinal quality cannot be discounted as an ingredient in plant food. Among the plants which stud the pasture on the Frontier, there are *Cluytia hirsuta*, the antidote for milt-ziekte, *Teucrium Africanum*, another anti-bacterial plant, *Stobaea speciosa*, a plant with a notable leaf, found on the Katberg, *Stobaea heterophylla* a thistle-like plant, *Sebaea crassulaefolia* and other species of the Gentian family; and many plants besides. The plants contain the alkaloids of the quinine group and other important principles, and they are distributed so uniformly and persistently, that they cannot be, and are not, avoided by the graminivora as plant-food, and as little can they be supposed to be where they are without serving an important purpose. It is noticeable, that they are more plentiful in what is called in this country the sour veldt, which consists of ranker grasses. They are perhaps more wanted there. It is possible the same thing may on a closer examination be found in the English natural pastures—the dandelion is an example of such plants—but in a colder climate the thing is less necessary.

APPENDIX VI.

A CUPPING INSTRUMENT FOR SNAKE-BITE.

Snake poison is ascertained to be a definite chemical compound, perfectly stable and indestructible, except by anhydrous sulphuric acid, permanganate of potash, and partially by carbolic acid; in fact, by those few substances which decompose and destroy any organic chemical. Ammonia has no effect on it, for when the poison is mixed with ammonia and injected into the bodies of animals, it retains its energy unimpaired, though ammonia, especially taken internally, to some extent counteracts its effects.

There are two kinds of snake poison, the colubrine of the cobras, and the viperine of the vipers or adders. The former is chiefly a nerve poison, and produces paralysis of the respiratory nerves. It kills by causing carbonic acid poisoning, which is accompanied by convulsions. The viperine venom is both a nerve and a blood poison, the latter action being often the more dangerous of the two. The puff-adder is our best known viper.

As snake poison is of this stable indestructible character, according to the dictates of common sense the first consideration is to get it out of the body, whatever the value of antidotes may be. Dr. Wall, who at the instance of the Indian Government carried out the experiments of Sir Joseph Fayrer to more definite results, is of opinion that nothing will save life in persons bitten by Indian snakes, except making a cut across the site of the bite, and dissecting out the subcutaneous tissues in which the venom is lodged, a sixth of an inch or more beneath the surface. Our South African snakes are not quite so venomous, and no one but a skilled surgeon would venture on such cutting and carving. Another plan, therefore, seemed desirable. A good many cases have occurred where life has been saved by sucking out the venom with the mouth. This suction, however, is feeble, and is also highly dangerous if there happens to be any skin wound in the gums or mouth. The proper thing would be a strong cupping instrument. The ordinary cupping instrument is unsuitable from the glass being too wide at the mouth. It is also too dear for common use. That of S. Maw and Son, London, is 22s. to the trade, and the retail price would be at least 30s. It seemed to me that nothing would serve but an instrument prepared expressly for snake-bite, and sold at about half a guinea. I accordingly induced Mr. William Hume, a well-known scientific instrument maker, Lothian Steet, Edinburgh, to prepare such an instrument, giving him an exact description. He produced one which is thoroughly effective. The barrel is of brass about five inches long by $\frac{7}{8}$ inch wide, with double valves, and a bell-shaped glass $\frac{3}{8}$ inch wide at the mouth, and enlarged above so as to hold an ounce of blood. As this instrument was thought rather large for carrying in one's pocket, a shorter form was prepared with the barrel of the syringe $2\frac{1}{2}$ inches long, and another of 3 inches, but the same in all other respects. The suction is powerful in all. The instrument is sold in Edinburgh at 10s. 6d. The maker's profit on it is so small, that it does not admit of advertising. In fact, but for the philanthropic desire to save human life, Mr. Hume would not have undertaken to produce this cupping instrument. What with customs duty, carriage, and commission, it could hardly be sold for less than 15s. in this country, unless an importer were to order six dozen, in which case there would be a reduction of of 20 per cent., making the original cost of each instrument 8s. 5d. The most convenient way of procuring a single instrument is to get it by parcel-post. The price is very moderate, considering that snake-bite tinctures are sold at 8s. 6d. to 12s. 6d., and are suspected of not keeping.

Treatment of snake-bite. The thing to be done immediately on a person being bitten, is to cut off the circulation from the part so as to prevent the venom from being absorbed. The best bandage is an india-rubber band or tube, which should be wound firmly and a number of times round the limb at the part next above the bite. As this band fits itself to depressions, it is more effective than whip-cord, even were it made so tight as to cut into the flesh. A soft reim is the next best, but anything, even a handkerchief, should should be used in an emergency. The next thing is to probe the two fang punctures with a sharp penknife, or a lancet. Scarifying is a mistake. It merely removes the superficial blood, while the venom remains lodged in the tissues. The proper way is to open up the punctures so as to get down to the venom, and secure the sucking out of it and the envenomed blood. The probing done, the mouth of the cupping glass should be moistened and pressed down firmly over the wound so as to allow no air to get in at the edge of the glass, and the piston should be worked up and down. The flesh will be sucked in, and the glass will soon be filled with blood. This may be repeated. If the cupping is performed before the poison has gone into the circulation, there is every reason to expect that life will be saved. It may be so, even if all the poison is not removed, for snake poison does not kill unless it goes above a certain proportion to the entire quantity of blood in the body. The plant antidote, described in Chapter IV., which should be administered at the first, may now be applied to the wound for absorption after washing it with Condy's fluid (a solution of permanganate of potash), if it is at hand.

P

Directions for using the Cupping instrument.—The instrument should be kept in a place known to all the household, and ready for immediate use. To keep it in perfect order, it should be examined periodically. In testing it, apply it to the chin or any fleshy part. If does not work, that may be from want of oiling the piston, or because the valves are wrong. The oil to use is sweet or olive oil, or else an animal oil, quite free from acid so as not to corrode the brass. As oil dries up, the oiling requires to be repeated now and again.

To reach the valves, unscrew the milled edge at the lower end of the syringe for the one valve, and screw off the bottom plate of the piston for the other. The valves may require simply to be wiped from oil or dirt. If a valve requires renewal, that is a very simple matter. It is merely a strip of oiled silk (the umbrella article, or that sold by druggists will do) put over a small hole, with its ends tied over a groove in the brass by means of a thread. The packing of the piston can also be easily renewed. In the larger barrel it consists of a round piece of leather, steeped in sweet oil, with a hole in the middle through which the screw of the bottom piston-plate passes and the sides are then folded up—an arrangement easily understood on inspection. With the shorter barrel, the packing of the piston consists of a few leather rings. The instrument is practically indestructible, and as all are made alike, glasses and other parts for that matter, could be replaced.

The original sample instrument in my possession was shown to the Premier, Sir J. Gordon Sprigg, and as he approved of it, he sent an order Home for six dozen, which were distributed for the use of Magistrates and District Surgeons. No farm-house should be without a cupping instrument for snake-bite; puff-adders and other snakes are so numerous, and there are so many children, servants, cattle, horses, and dogs liable to be bitten. The cupping glass will also be serviceable for the sting of the scorpion, the bite of the tarantula, the stings of wasps, and if applied at the moment, for poisonous blood or matter getting into a cut or scratch, or for sucking out the venom introduced by the bite of a mad dog.

APPENDIX VII.

STRYCHNINE IN SNAKE-BITE.

An extract from an Article in the *Australasian Medical Gazette* will show the Australian mode of treating snake-bite with strychnine:—

"The merits of the treatment of snake-bite by the hypodermic injection of strychnia, as suggested by Dr. Müller, of Yackandandah, Victoria, have now been so thoroughly proved by the experience of practitioners in all parts of Australia and Tasmania, that it is a matter for surprise that it is not used in every case showing serious symptoms. A number of instances have been recently reported in the lay press of the various colonies of death following on snake-bite where strychnia had not been used, but in which the persons treating them depended on the supposed remedial effects of ammonia and alcohol, both of which my own experience has led me to have no faith in. In fact I believe alcohol to be positively injurious, whilst the liability of ammonia to produce phlegmonous inflammation when injected subcutaneously is a subject for serious consideration independently of its very questionable utility in snake-poisoning. With the cases recorded in this journal of the invariably good results following the strychnine treatment when properly carried out, I do not hesitate to say that, in my opinion, the life of any patient who dies from the effects of snake-poison, who has not been treated with adequate doses of strychnia, has been sacrificed to ignorance or prejudice. Independently of the authority of Dr. Müller, as set forth in his Paper read before the Melbourne Medical Congress in January, 1889, which, however, was most culpably omitted from the Transactions, but published in the *Australasian Medical Gazette* for April, 1890, the cases reported at the same time by Dr. Thwaites, of Tallangatta, Victoria, who said that he adopted the treatment on the authority of Dr. Müller, in one of which he injected first 10 minims, then 20 minims, and finally of 15 minims of liquor strychniae B.P., with resulting recovery; in the other, a girl of thirteen, who was apparently moribund, he gave a single dose of 17 minims, which proved absolutely effective and apparently snatched her from the jaws of death—show how efficient adequate doses of strychnia are. . . . . . .

In the No. for February last, Dr. Ray, of Seymour, Victoria, says that on December 30, 1890, he treated a man bitten by a tiger snake *(Hoplocephalus curtus)*, and that during six hours he injected subcutaneously $\frac{2}{5}$ grain of strychnia in addition to a considerable quantity given by the mouth. He says: 'No further difficulty was experienced in keeping the patient awake, and after slight twitching of the hands occurred, the drug was stopped, and the patient made a good recovery.' He also adds: 'The most satisfactory feature of the case was the unmistakeable effect of the drug in counteracting the effect of the snake-venom, every dose after the second having a distinct effect within three or four minutes, lasting from half to one-and-a-half hours before the tendency to coma returned. Only two small doses of brandy of one ounce each were given after the treatment commenced, one three hours after, and another at night.'

In the same issue Dr. Forbes, of Charters Towers, Queensland, reports the case of a boy of six years of age bitten by a snake, which was killed and identified as a *death adder (Acanthophis Antarctica)*. He says that at 9 p.m. the father rushed in saying his boy was dead, and indeed his statement seemed too true. The child was lying quite limp, face blue, eyes half shut, extremities cold, no pulse perceptible, no respiration visible. I at once injected 10 minims Liq. strychniae B.P., and did artificial respiration. He soon began to improve, and in about 20 minutes he was able to speak. He was watched all night, but suffered no relapse, and was discharged next day.

In the same No., Dr. Weekes, of Lithgow, New South Wales, writing of three cases of snake-bite, says:—" These patients were all comatose, exhibiting all the usual symptoms of snake-bite poisoning, and in one, my last case, the patient had convulsions. In all, I gave hypodermic injections of Liq. strychniae B.P. minims XV., and the effect was most marked, the patient being completely roused and becoming quite sensible and rational each time. In my last case, that of a woman, the first injection of minims XV. roused her a little, but not completely. In 20 minutes I gave her another of the same amount, and in 10 minutes she awoke and asked to be allowed to walk about herself, and from this time she made a good recovery. . .

I have quoted the above cases as conclusively showing that patients severely suffering from the effects of snake-poison require what would otherwise prove lethal doses of strychnia to ensure their recovery, and that the weak point in the treatment of snake-bite by this means has frequently been the hesitancy with which such doses have been used in critical cases. I again express my opinion, published on previous occasions, that every effort should be made to eliminate the venom previous to its absorption, by the excision of the bite : that no alcohol should be given or ammonia administered either by the mouth or beneath the skin, and that the patient's strength should not be exhausted by violent exercise, or by the infliction of various tortures, (including in more than one instance the playing of 'the town band,' whose aid had been obtained in desperate cases of snake-poison as being absolutely antagonistic to mental quietude), and that only when the toxic symptoms of the bite arise should strychnia be administered. Directly they appear $\frac{1}{10}$ of a grain should be injected hypodermically, or even $\frac{1}{6}$ if the insensibility is very marked. This dose should be repeated in 20 minutes if coma or collapse continues. If the two doses are insufficient, more must be given at frequent intervals as required either by the persistence or recurrence of insensibility. The injections may be safely given until twitchings of the muscles show that the physiological action of strychnia has been brought about, when the administration should be suspended until they disappear. They may be renewed if symptoms come on which show more of the remedy is required to assure the patient's safety. . . . .

We have not yet heard whether this treatment has been used in cases of bites by Indian snakes, of which Sir Joseph Fayrer, in a letter to myself commenting on a suggestion I made at a meeting of the New South Wales Branch of the British Medical Association in 1887, and also in a Paper read before the Adelaide Medical Congress in 1887, that possibly the inhalation of ether might have a good effect, says: "I think it possible that the mode of treatment you suggest might be of use in cases where only a limited dose of the poison had been inoculated, but I fear in cases where a full dose of cobra poison has entered the circulation that we can do little if anything towards arresting a fatal result." Experiments on dogs were made by Sir Joseph, and also by Dr. Vincent Richards many years since, with a view of determining the utility of the hypodermic injection of strychnia in Indian snake-bite, and the conclusion they arrived at by their tests on these animals was unfavourable. On reading the report of the experiments I was struck with the tolerance exhibited by the dogs of the *very* large doses of strychnia exhibited, some of whom recovered from injections of cobra poison which had proved fatal to similar animals, and from quantities of strychnia which I believe would have been certainly fatal but for the counteracting effect of the snake venom. Dr. Müller is of opinion that experiments on the lower animals are not satisfactory as showing the effect of strychnia administered for snake poison to human beings, and that the only evidence which is conclusive is the result of its administration to men and women who have been bitten. The result of the cases I have quoted in the earlier portion of this article, when compared with the tests on dogs by Sir Joseph Fayrer and Dr. Vincent Richards, goes to support this view, though of course it is possible that the effects of the poison of the Indian snakes is sufficiently different from those of this continent to make that of strychnia on the human subject different to what has been found to follow its use for the treatment of poisoning by snakes in this country.

However, with the general knowledge—confirmed unhesitatingly by that high authority Sir Joseph Fayrer—that an effective bite by a cobra is invariably fatal, the use of full doses of strychnia in such cases is not a hazardous experiment, which even if it left the victim unbenefited, would not add to his danger of death. Under these circumstances I can only hope that medical practitioners in India, on the evidence of the remarkable success of the remedy in Australia, will use the hypodermic injection of strychnia in cases of poisoning by the snakes of that country, and carefully record the result. I may say that had I the opportunity, I should unhesitatingly make use of it for cobra bite myself, and should use doses of $\frac{1}{5}$ to $\frac{1}{4}$ of a grain to commence with, modifying subsequent doses as the exigences of the symptoms required. Should this meet the eye of any medical man in India who has used the remedy on the human subject, I shall esteem it a great favour if he will communicate particulars of the doses administered, with the result, to me as Editor of the *Australasian Medical Gazette*, for publication."

J. MILDRED CREED, L.R.C.P., M.R.C.S.E.

APPENDIX VIII.

MESEMBRYANTHEMUM TUBERS AS FERMENTS.

The tubers of several species belonging to the Mesembryanthemum Family are employed in this country as ferments in making bread or mead, for anything in fact requiring fermentation. To prepare the tubers for use, they dry them after removing the cuticle, and reduce them to a powder, the action of which is extremely rapid, and it occasions no sour fermentation. This mode of fermenting is employed in the lower Fish River and Keiskama valleys, and elsewhere. The domestic importance of such ferments is evident enough, when sour bread made with sour dough is the common rule. Dr. J. B. Slater has been investigating the subject, and thinks that this fermenting property runs through the whole Mesembryanthemum Family, and that the tubers might be made a great export. Whether it be the case or not, that the property is universal in this Family, we may infer from the analogy of Medicinal plants that there are a few species much more valuable than the others. Which these are could most easily be found from noting those that have actually come into use.

It is supposed that the imported yeast-cakes so called are prepared from mesembryanthemum tubers. If so, it is surely a piece of extravagance to import such things into the country *par excellence* of this great Order.

APPENDIX IX.

SNAKE-POISON AS A PROPHYLACTIC.

Natives of various races think that swallowing snake-poison prevents the deadly effects of snake-bite. Several things give plausibility to this opinion—its general acceptance; cases in proof; and the circumstance that venomous snakes are not killed by the bite of venomous snakes, as harmless serpents are.

Popular belief is always worth something, and the fact that persons who have swallowed snake-poison attack dangerous snakes in the most venturesome manner on the strength of that opinion is sufficient proof of confidence in it.

There are also cases in evidence. An English farmer near the lower Keiskama, too highly educated to be readily imposed on, mentions the statements of his native herd, who says 'that he swallows the venom from the poison-bag of the puff-adder every year, and after that, so far from being afraid of snakes, he plays with puff-adders.' He had been bitten by a puff-adder, and showed his master the marks of the fangs on his wrist, but he suffered no serious injury from being protected in the manner stated. He feels very strange and confused, he says, for two or three days after swallowing the poison, and cannot do anything. A case bringing out another phase of the question was that of a Colonist near Queenstown, who was bitten in the arm by a puff-adder while lifting sheaves in the harvest field. A Bushman extracted the poison-bag, and made him swallow the poison, but whether that was meant to be of service then or only for the future, does not appear. The Bushman told him not to slaughter animals while the poison remained in his blood, else the meat would putrefy. Some time afterwards he went into Kaffirland, and was asked by a farmer to slaughter pigs. When he told what the Bushman said, the farmer simply laughed at him, and he accordingly consented, with the result that the carcases became tainted and useless. The quantity of poison in the blood that would come from his hands could only be small, and the action must therefore have been from something that multiplies rapidly, and not from a mere chemical. This putrefying action of snake-poison suggests the use of antiseptics in snake-bite by the puff-adder especially, besides the use of a nerve stimulant such as strychnia.

Venomous snakes, in numerous instances at least, are not fatally affected by a bite from their own, or from any other venomous species, and it is affirmed that their blood is poisonous, no doubt from the venom going through it, and that may be the circumstance which gives them immunity. The analogy of other poisons, such as arsenic and laudanum, gives countenance to this, for persons taking small doses can bear on an occasion an amount which would kill anyone else.

After all, swallowing snake-poison as a prophylactic is a precarious experiment. The poison certainly is not so dangerous in the stomach as in the blood, but what if there were some lesion or raw spot on the mucous membrane, where it might be absorbed?

Snake-poison could however be taken with safety in homœopathic doses, and by going on for some time, it would have all the effect of a single large dose. It is nothing new in medicine to employ snake-poison in the cure of disease.

Since this was written, I received an Abstract of a Paper communicated by Professor Thomas R. Fraser, LL.D., to the Royal Society of Edinburgh, on rendering Animals immune against the venom of serpents; and on the Antidotal Properties of the Blood-serum of the immunized animals.

As this series of highly important experiments is not yet completed, it will be enough here to indicate the lines along which they were conducted. Professor Fraser proceeded on the idea, for which he produced a wide consensus of opinion, that venom in the blood, or certain effects on the blood produced by it, is the circumstance that protects venomous snakes, and persons who had swallowed snake-poison or who had recovered after being bitten, from the otherwise fatal effects of snake-bite, and setting out from that, he introduced snake-poison by subcutaneous injection into numerous animals—the guinea-pig, rabbit, white rat, cat, grass snake, and also the horse—in gradually increasing doses, beginning with one non-lethal, with the result that they could be brought on to bear in a single dose what would have killed two, four, or five animals of the same weight and species, had they been unprotected, and in one case enough for fifty such, the total quantity of venom injected in that instance in the course of five or six months being capable of killing 370 animals of the same species. During the process of immunization, the animals increased in weight, they fed well, and appeared to acquire increased vigour and liveliness. This was frequently exemplified in the smaller animals, such as rabbits; and also, very conspicuously, in an aged and previously sedate horse, which in the process of immunization, received eleven times the estimated minimum-lethal dose.

The next step was to test by experiment what power the blood-serum of such venom-proof animals (he names it *antivenene*) had when dissolved in water and injected subcutaneously, to arrest the progress of snake-poison introduced into the bodies of animals. Four series of experiments were made on rabbits—

1 In one series, the venom was mixed outside of the body with the antivenene, and immediately thereafter the mixture was injected under the skin of the animal.

2 In the second series, the venom and the antivenene were almost simultaneously injected into opposite sides of the body.

3 In the third series, the antivenene was injected some considerable time before the venom.

4 In the fourth series, the venom was first injected, and thirty minutes afterwards the antivenene.

In the First series, the exact quantity of antivenene required to neutralize the effects of a minimum-lethal dose of the venom was ascertained, and was found to range from $\frac{1}{2}$ to $\frac{1}{250}$ of a cubic centimetre (15.43 minims) for each kilogramme ($2\frac{1}{5}$ ℔s) of the animal's weight—a very small amount.

In the Fourth series, important as involving the recovery of persons bitten, otherwise fatally, death was prevented by the injection of 1.5, 1, and .8 cubic centimetres of the antivenene *thirty minutes* after a minimum-lethal dose of the venom had been injected; but a less amount .75 c.c. was insufficient to prevent death; and with a double minimum-lethal dose of the venom 5 c.c. per kilogramme prevented death. Indications were also obtained that probably death may be prevented by several administrations of antivenene, rather than one, and by introducing it near the bitten spot rather than in distant parts.

In a subsequent communication to the Royal Society, Dr. Fraser stated, that the blood-serum of the horse furnished a much more powerful antivenene than that of rabbits, and he expressed a belief that antivenene might yet be supplied from the blood-serum of venomous serpents.

It is unnecessary to say more on the subject at present, as the experimentation is not concluded; but we are apparently now within sight of a reliable antidote for snakebite. South African experience affords a corroboration of the principle on which it proceeds, for there are cases of experts applying to a poisonous bite the flesh of the venomous snake with its blood and lymph to arrest the action of the venom on the person bitten.

The use of antivenene or strychnine ought not to supersede cupping to remove the poison from a bite, nor even the employment of certain antidotes especially antiseptics, were it only to prevent local mischief. In saving human life, nothing should be left open to chance.

APPENDIX X.

MUSHROOMS

The common edible mushroom, Kaffir, *in-Kowane*, is plentiful in many parts of this country. It comes up with the early Spring rains before other Fungi, and is distinguishable from its globular form at first, its very white colour, and its pink gills. It is not to be used after the pink turns brown, or black. No notice of mushrooms would be required here, but for the scarcely known fact that the genuine mushroom is poisonous when it grows on rotten wood or on any decaying matter. Some time ago a distinguished evangelist, a member of the McAll Mission in Paris, had gone with his family to the country for a short rest, and a domestic gathered mushrooms, which were duly examined and were found to be all of the right kind. On their being eaten, however, the whole family were poisoned, though he alone died. This sad result was traced to some of the mushrooms being gathered off decaying wood.

There is a very large white mushroom *(i-Kowe)* which is eaten by the Kaffirs. For some reason or other, they regard the former as poisonous.

APPENDIX XI.

FRICTION.

The form of treatment called *massage* requires no notice here as being well known; but the value of friction to prevent indigestion, acidity, sleeplessness, torpid action of the liver and bowels, and weak action of the heart is hardly known. The kind of friction meant is that with a horse-hair friction glove which has a short pile like a brush. (The sort made by Dinneford & Co., London, is recommended.) This friction should be over the great sympathetic nerve, the stomach, the liver, and the viscera, and there is also a horse-hair friction strap for the spine. As the action referred to is to stimulate the nervous system—not intended to keep the skin pure, or to bring the blood to the surface, though it does that also—it should be long continued, for a quarter of an hour at least, and ought to be light so as not to irritate the skin, which would be of no benefit for the object designed.

This sort of friction increases the force of the pulsation, and of the peristaltic action, and causes a flow of the gastric juice, the bile, and the secretions generally. It also remedies the minor derangements, such as acidity or flatulence, occasioned by the use of Tonics and blood-purifiers.

APPENDIX XII.

WOUNDS AND SORES.

The common thick-leafed *Prickly Pear* stands almost alone in the rapidity with which it draws sores, and brings boils and hard swellings to the point of suppuration. In preparing the leaf, remove the skin from one side of it, and heat the portion of the leaf taken in an oven, or at a fire till it becomes quite soft. The fleshy side should then be applied as hot as it can be borne, and when it cools, the same process should be repeated till the desired result is obtained.

The effect of the leaf in extracting thorns is still more remarkable. In a case where a prickly-pear thorn had become deeply imbedded in the foot from treading on it, this remedy was resorted to after all the attempts and appliances of a doctor to extract the thorn had failed. The heated leaf was applied and renewed many times in succession during the course of a day, with the result that the head of the thorn came up a little, and the thorn was then gently and easily drawn out. It proved to be an inch long. Heating the plant substance in these appliances to wounds and sores is highly important, but the constant hot repetition is necessary only in urgent cases. A trader in Tembuland states that a Kaffir expert there has an appliance which makes an obstinate thorn drop out, and that he offered him a sum of money to reveal the secret, but he declined to do so. It is probably just this, or one exactly on the same principle, but if the remedy is as good, it cannot be better than this.

APPENDIX XIII.

A RESPIRATOR OR INHALER.

Respirators or Inhalers are costly, uselessly so. A simple and effective inhaler can be made by cutting with common scissors out of a sheet of perforated zinc with fine bores, a piece six inches by four, or it may be made smaller if wished. This is folded into a wide-mouthed conical pocket by making the middle point of the longer or 6 inch edge the apex of the cone, and bending round the two 3 inch parts to meet with an overlap at the top; where they are stitched together through the bores. A white silk ribbon binding is then put round the wide mouth, and linen tapes are attached to the projecting angles, to tie above the ears. A piece of wetted sponge with some crystallized carbolic acid in the heart of it is then put into the bottom of the conical pocket, and the inhaler can be worn for a short time before going to bed—preferably then as it tends to induce a slight perspiration—either to include the nostrils or not. It is not easy to give the exact quantity of carbolic acid. One part to twenty of water is the proportion with a close inhaler; but as the carbolic vapour is in this case diluted with air coming in at the sides of the respirator, the crystals can be used in a larger proportion, only care should be taken that no pain is caused, but merely a sweet sensation on the palate. Carbolic acid has a wonderful virtue in nipping in the bud consumptive germs which may have entered through breathing. It also allays bronchial inflammation, and stops an incessant cough. In some cases, however, it proves unsuitable and produces unfavourable symptoms, and its use ought therefore to be experimental and tentative.

This inhaler, which will cost a mere trifle, can be empolyed also with eucalyptol, thymol, and oil of peppermint, and it is of great service to use it, especially with carbolic acid, when one has to go into an atmosphere poisoned with germs or with noxious smells. The carbolized sponge is perfectly effective though dry, if one breathe hot air out through it, as well as draw air in, since the dry acid easily becomes vaporized.

APPENDIX XIV.

DRUGS FOR EXPORT.

From the South African Flora there are only two drugs of any consequence exported, buchu and aloes, though there is a large number of real medicinal plants employed, not indeed by the highly conservative medical practitioners, who are mostly educated in Europe, but by people in general and by Native specialists. For export, we may throw out the major portion of these plants as not fitted to supersede the plant resources of the pharmacopoeia, which are selected products from every clime, but there remain ten or twelve, which either fill a place left blank in the regular course of medicine, or which would prove important auxiliaries or substitutes.

For anthrax there are two important Acanthaceous plants, *Blepharis Capensis* and *Crabbea cirsioides*, and with them must be joined the Euphorbiaceous *Cluytia hirsuta*, which last in combination with either of the former has been highly efficacious in curing Malignant pustule, and other forms of blood-poisoning. The Kaffir mode of treatment is also too rational and successful to be neglected. *Cluytia* is fitted besides to nip these maladies in the bud, and it would probably act as a prophylactic to ward off wool-sorter's disease.

Among blood-purifiers *Bulbine latifolia* or *alöoides* holds a conspicuous place. It removes the lactic acid or other impurity remaining after rheumatic fever, as has been proved in numerous cases. But it appears also to arrest degeneration in the involuntary muscles, the heart and others, or even to retrieve it, whether proceeding from this fever, or from cholera and influenza. That has yet to be thoroughly tested. If it turns out to do so, it would hardly be possible to exaggerate the importance of this drug.

Sutherlandia frutescens, R. Br. has for its proper function the cure of dysenteric diarrhoea, and nervous dyspepsia. Its leaves are intensely bitter. This shrub has been put forward as a cancer cure from its efficacy in healing gangrenous sores, but those who do so are not familiar with the characteristic marks of typical cancer, and when tried in that it has failed. A mistake made in its proper use as a drug does not invalidate its claims otherwise.

Lasiosiphon Meisneri. There are sores and eruptions which defy every effort to heal them on account of an impurity of blood behind them. A tincture made from the roots of this plant, taken internally, has a singular power in healing sores and eruptions by removing this impurity. An incurable sore goes on poisoning the blood, and many blood-purifiers, however excellent for their proper objects, fail to affect it. The principle in the root is volatile.

Heteromorpha arborescens, and *Bulbine asphodeloides*. The white inner root-bark of the former and the tubers of the other are antidotes for scrofula. Dr. Koch, the discoverer of the *bacillus tuberculosis*, maintains that scrofula of every kind proceeds from the bacillus which is the cause of consumption; and others now insist that the bacillus cannot have been communicated hereditarily, since consumption does not develop much before the age of twenty, but only a pre-disposition or some degeneration fitted to nurture the bacillus which is acquired casually. If we suppose this to be the case, something might be done earlier to remove the scrofulous taint and thus prevent the accession of the bacillus, and as there is a limit to the employment of iodine of which cod-liver oil is the vehicle, other drugs might be employed to remove the taint, and the capabilities of Heteromorpha and of this Bulbine ought therefore to be tested experimentally.

Cissampelos Capensis, Davidjes. This potent drug is used as a stomach and liver medicine, and as a tonic, in all which it may do some good and probably more harm. The really valuable use of the root is for syphilitic blood-poisoning, in which a tincture is of extreme value as a blood-purifier. It may be employed as an auxiliary to mercury, or as a substitute in cases where mercury is contra-indicated. Possibly some of its valuable applications have yet to be found out. It is probably poisonous, and care must be taken in the quantity of the dose.

Monsonia ovata. An infusion of this plant of the Geranium Family, including the roots, is a specific for certain forms of chronic dysentery and diarrhoea. As a sedative and mild astringent it acts best where the malady is an inflamed state of the mucous membrane of the bowels and also of the stomach. It is suprising that a plant which has such a repute in this country has not been exported to England long ere now.

The whole of these plants deserve to be thoroughly tested by physicians in South Africa and at Home to find out what they are really capable of, and their being so largely used in this country affords a presumption that they are important.

Besides drugs, there is a South African beetle which ought to be exported for blistering purposes.

The Spanish blistering fly, *Cantharis vesicatoria*, a green beetle with a coppery gloss, is likely to be superseded in certain markets by a South African one, *Mylabris bifasciata*, a black beetle with yellow stripes, which yields more than twice as much *cantharidin*, and is therefore of double the value, provided this species can be found in sufficient quantity.

A special interest attaches to the species M. bifasciata on account of its economic value. A comparison between it and the Spanish fly will show its superiority. This Mylabris yields 2·09 per cent. of *cantharidin*, accompanied with only 10·45 per cent. of extractive, while the Spanish Cantharis produces only ·42 per cent. and the more troublesome amount of 18 per cent. of extractive. A London expert, who was asked to report on the former, laughed at the idea of there being any blistering properties in it, and made a test on his right arm, which raised such a beautiful blister that he was unable to write his report.

The distinctive mark of M. bifasciata is its having two, and only two, dark ochre-yellow bars across the elytra or wing-covers, the one behind being edged with a rufous border. Compared with this, M. lunata has three bars with the last two much more sinuate or waved than those of the other species. The front one, which is just where the elytra are jointed to the body, consists of a curve on each wing-cover, so that when these are closed, the two curves form together a semilunar bar with the concave side forwards. The antennæ of M. bifasciata are in bead-form, getting thicker toward the tip, and consist of 11 joints, the two at the base being black, and the rest yellow. Those of M. lunata have the four at the base black, and the rest ochre-brown. The entire length of M. bifasciata is from ·787 to ·984 of an inch. M. Lunata is rather smaller, from ·55 to ·708 of an inch. If the valuable species is collected for export, Messrs Hale and Son, the drug brokers of 10, Fenchurch Avenue, London, recommend that it should be made up in tin or zinc-lined cases, soldered to be air-tight, each to contain a cwt. There is a danger that the beetles may be eaten up by insects, in which case the sale is forced, and the price may be only 2s. 3d. a ℔. At best it may be 7s. 6d. a ℔. The price paid here for collecting should not exceed a 1s. a ℔., and it is of no use to send any other species to the London market.

Mylabris, like Cantharis, is a genus of the family Cantharidæ, and is fully represented here, though there is but one species in Europe. The species in this country have been called Sergeant beetles from the yellow stripes across their wing-covers. If there is a field of peas in bloom, they come in numbers to devour the blossoms and when there is a garden of roses, they alight there and eat the petals down to the very receptacle, so that roses cannot be got between the first hot breath of summer when the beetles arrive and the cold gusts of autumn when they depart. They are above such coarse fare as zinnias and balsams, if they can get anything better. They shorten to half a day the single day of life which nature gives to the gorgeous tiger iris.

Note on Exportation.—In preparing *Cluytia* for export—the short kind found growing in the veldt is much the best—the leafy twigs should be dried rapidly, after being shortly under pressure, else they will be of an off-colour, and will crumble in being closely packed. The same applies to *Monsonia, Blepharis, Sutherlandia*, and any other plant with leaves. With *Bulbine alöoides*, the tubers require to be thoroughly dried with artificial heat or by the sun, else they will become sour or mouldy. The larger tubers must be sliced. In *Lasiosiphon, isi-Dikili,* the active principle is so volatile, that the root soon becomes inert. Probably it would be preferable with this valuable root to make a tincture while it is quite fresh, and export that. If a tincture of a fine red tint without muddiness is wished from *isi-Dikili*, and a similar one of a sherry colour from *Davidjes*, the outer brown cortex should be scraped off.

INDEX OF BOTANICAL NAMES.

[*The more important plants are put in Italics.*]

Acocanthera venenata,	8, 37, 45	Cissampelos Pareira,	..	143
Acocanthera spectabilis,	8, 37, 45	Cissampelos torulosa,	..	143
Agapanthus, ...	147	Clematis brachiata, Thun.	101,	161
Agrimonia Eupatoria, Lin. var. Capensis, Harv.	108	Cluytia, ...		165
		Cluytia hirsuta,	8, 48, 56, 63	155
Alepidea Amatymbica, E. and Z.	67	Cluytia pulchella, Müll.	..	171
Alepidea ciliaris, ...	67	Conyza ivaefolia, Less.	..	154
Aloe ferox, var. supralaevis,	120	Convolvulus, ...		174
Aloe saponaria, or latifolia,	73, 133	*Cotyledon orbiculata*,	..	128
Aloe tenuior, Harv... ..	105	*Crabbea cirsioides*, 8, 35, 45, 55,		123
Amygdalis Persica, ...	79, 165	Cucumis Africanus, Lin.	..	177
Andropogon, ...	182	Cyperus, ...		63
Anemone Caffra, E. and Z.	121			
Artemisia Afra, Jacq. ..	95	Datura stramonium, Lin.	..	123
Asparagus stipulaceus, var. spinescens, 183.		Dianthus, ...		147
		Dicoma anomala, ..	.. 64,	155
Athrixia heterophylla, Less.	122			
Atropa belladonna, ...	149	Ehretia Zeyheriana,	..	171
		Elaeodendron croceum,	..	178
Blepharis Capensis, 8, 35, 45,48, 55, 123, 140		Emex spinosa, Campd.	.. 70,	168
		Eriosema salignum, E. Mey.	90,	134
Brachylaena elliptica,	126, 169	Erithrina Humei, E. Mey	..	90
Bulbine alöoides, and *B. latifolia*, 135	84,	Eucalyptus globulus,	..	95
		Euclea lanceolata, ..	..	119
Bulbine asphodeloides, Schult.	89, 130	Euphorbia, ...		136
Buphane toxicaria, ..	158, 180	Euphorbia bupleurifolia, Jacq.		119, 137
Calla Aethiopica, ...	78	Euphorbia pugniformis,	119,	137
Calophanes Persoonii, ..	41	Exomis axyrioides, Fenzl. ..		131
Cannabis sativa, ...	28, 164			
Capparis citrifolia, ...	156	Ficus Capensis, Thun.	..	169
Cassia mimosoides, Lin. ..	118			
Chaenostoma rotundifolium,	112	Gazania pinnata, var. integrifolia, 141, 178		
Chaetacanthus Persoonii, T. Anders.	41			
Chenopodium ambrosioides, Lin.	173	Gnidia, ...		127
Chenopodium vulvaria, Lin.	129	Grewia occidentalis, Lin. ..		171
Chloris compressa, Nees ..	102	Gunnera perpensa, Lin. ..		161
Chlorophytum comosum, Baker	140			
Cissampelos Capensis, 43, 45, 86, 143		Haplocarpha lyrata Harv.		179

INDEX OF BOTANICAL NAMES.

Hartwegia comosa, Nees . . 140
Helichrysum appendiculatum, Less. 101
Helichrysum nudiflorum, Less. 100
Hermannia candicans, Ait. . . 134
Heteromorpha arborescens, Cham. and Schl 71, 86, 87, 168
Hibiscus aethiopicus, Lin. . . 75
Hibiscus pusillus, ... 76
Hibiscus Trionum, Lin. . . 76, 131
Hippobromus alata, E. and Z. 112
Hypoxis obliqua, . . 167, 175
Hypoxis sericea, . . 167, 174

Imantophyllum miniatum, Hook. 44
Indigofera patens, E. and Z. 68, 125
Indigofera Zeyheri, Spreng. 69

Lantana salviaefolia, Jacq. 3, 111
Lasiosiphon anthylloides, . . 36
Lasiosiphon linifolius, . . 36, 127
Lasiosiphon Meisneri, 35, 45, 77, 86 125
Lasiospermum radiatum, Trev. 182
Leonotis leonurus 8, 20, 25, 27, 45, 103, 106
Leonotis ovata, 8, 20, 25, 29, 45, 155
Lichtensteinia interrupta, E. Mey. 98
Lippia asperifolia, Rich. . . 59, 101
Lithospermum, ... 147

Mahernia chrysantha, Planch. 70
Malva parviflora, Lin. . . 74
Matricaria globifera, . . 92
Matricaria nigellaefolia, DC. 58, 147
Melianthus comosus, Vahl 32, 83
Mesembryanthemum bellidiflorum, 183
Mesembryanthemum micranthum, Harv. 182
Monsonia ovata, 3, 45, 48, 97
Myaris inaequalis, Presl. 160, 179

Noltea Africana, Reich. . . 157

Oxalis Smithii, Sond. . . 107

Panicum sanguinale, . . 102
Parmelia conspersa, . . 41
Pelargonium alchemilloides, Willd. 74
Pelargonium pulverulentum, Colv. 168, 170
Pelargonium ramosissimum, Willd. 100
Pelargonium reniforme, Curt. 81, 115, 168
Pellaea hastata, ... 102
Pentanisia variabilis, Harv. 65, 90
Petroselinum sativum, . . 134
Phytolacca stricta, . . 151, 177
Pittosporum viridiflorum, Sims 156
Plantago 82
Plumbago 148
Polygala serpentaria, E. and Z. 44
Polygonum tomentosum, var. glabrum, 156
Pterocelastrus variabilis, Sond. 175

Ranunculus Capensis, 70, 102, 165
Ranunculus pinnatus, . . 70, 102
Rhyncosia gibba, E. Mey. . . 90
Richardia Africana, . . 78
Ricinus communis, Lin. . . 123
Rubia petiolaris, DC. . . 89, 117
Rumex Eckloni, ... 107

Salix Capensis, ... 94
Salvia scabia, Thun. . . 141
Samolus Valerandi, Lin. . . 148
Sansevieria thyrsiflora, . . 109
Sarcostemma viminale, E. Mey. 159
Scabiosa columbaria, Lin. . . 113
Schistostephium flabelliforme, Less. 103
Scilla lancedifolia, ... 155
Sebaea crassulaefolia, 42, 45, 147
Senecio angulatus, ... 180
Senecio concolor, DC. . . 83
Senecio deltoides, Less. . . 113
Senecio latifolius, var. barbellatus, 82
Sideroxylon inerme, Lin. . . 155

INDEX OF BOTANICAL NAMES.

Silene Burchellii, Ott.	89	Urtica,	.. 82, 113
Solanum Capense, 91, 100, 117, 124, 134, 160		Venidium arctotoides Less.	81
Solanum melongena,	144	Viscum,	176
Solanum nigrum, Lin.	59, 133		
Solanum Sodomaeum,	130	Withania somnifera, Dun. 50, 59, 83, 100, 133, 145, 157, 166	
Sutherlandia frutescens, R. Br. 62, 66, 86, 116, 138			
		Xanthoxylon Capense. Harv. 44, 58, 126	
Teucrium Africanum, 20, 30, 59, 62			
Thunbergia Capensis, Thun.	91	Xysmalobium lapathifolium,	61, 80
Toxicophloea Thunbergii, Harv. 8, 37, 45		Zizyphus mucronata, Willd.	88, 136

INDEX OF KAFFIR PLANT-NAMES.

um- Bangandlela,	71, 86, 87, 168	um- Fisi,		.. 90, 134
um- Belebele,	 159	um- Fiyo,		 171
im- Bikicane,	.. 129, 173			
um- Bomvane,	 178	in- Geelwane,		73, 84, 133, 135
u- Boqo,	 174	um- Geunube,		 94
ili- Bulawa,	.. .. 42, 147	i- Gqita, ..		 97
um- Bungushe,	 98	um- Gwali, ..		 97
isi- Cimamlilo,	.. .. 65, 90	um- Hlaba, ..		 120
i- Colocolo,	 100	um- Hlahlampetu,		 173
in- Cwadi,	.. .. 158, 180	um- Hlambezo,		 146
isi- Cwe, ..	 81	um- Hlavutwa,		 123
		um- Hleli, ..		 171
um- Dambiso,	 83	um- Hlonhlo,		 136
in- Dawa,	 63	um- Hlonyane		 99
in- Dembu,	 176	um- Hlonyane womlambo,		.. . 58, 147
isi- Dikili,	.. 35, 77, 86, 125	ubu-Hlungu,		.. .. 30, 41
in- Dindilili,	 180	ubu-Hlungu be-Dila,		56, 63, 155
in- Dlebe yemvu,	.. 101	ubu-Hlungu besi-Gcawu,		35, 55, 123
ili- Dliso,	.. .. 65, 90	140		
i- Dolo lenkonyana,	.. 107	ubu-Hlungu be-Mamba,		.. 32, 44
isi- Duli, ..	.. 126, 169	ubu-Hlungu be-Nyoka,		.. 37
i- Dwara,	 82	ubu-Hlungu be-Nyushu		30, 59, 62
isi- Fikane,	.. 182	u- Jejune, ..	..	.. 140
um- Fincafincane,	.. 27, 106			

INDEX OF KAFFIR PLANT-NAMES.

i- Kalana,		105	u- Sikiki,		141
in- Kamamasane,		119, 137	um- Sintsana,		90
isi- Kolokoto,		109	um- Sobo,		59, 133
i- Kubalo lika Mlanjeni,		170	um- Sobosobo,		133
in- Kubele,		74	um- Solo womlambo,		147
in- Kunzane,		70, 168			
um- Kwenkwe,		156	u- Tangazana,		177
um- Kwinti,		141, 178	in- Telezi,		89
			um- Ti wamadoda,		148
ubu-Lembu belitye,		27, 41	in- Tlungunyembe,		37, 158
u- Luzi,		169	in- Tsema,		119, 133
u- Lwatile,		112	i- Tshongwe,		61, 80, 115
			i- Tshongwana,		161
u- Madolwana,		102	in- Tsihlo,		156, 178
um- Muncwane,		107	um- Tuma,		130, 144
			um- Tumana, 91, 100, 117, 124, 154,		
um- Ngana,		118	160		
u- Nomolwana,		74	i- Tyolo,		101, 161
um- Nqabaza,		171	u- Tywala bentaka,		111
um- Nquma,		109	i- Tywina		175
um- Nukambiba,		160, 179			
um- Nungumabele,		44, 58, 126	im- Vane,		183
um- Nyanja,		151, 177	ubu-Vumba, 50, 59, 83, 100, 133, 145		
in- Nyinga,		108	157, 166		
in- Nyongwane,		64, 155	um- Vumbangwe		123
um- Pafa,		88, 136	i- Xalanxa,		167, 174, 175
i- Palode,		157			
isi- Petshane,		103	um- Ya		28, 164
i- Pewula,		128	i- Yeza lesi-Diya,		157
i- Puzi lomlambo,		161	i- Yeza lam-Ehlo,		113
			i- Yeza lo-Gezo,		122
i- Qina,		182	i- Yeza le-Hashe,		89, 91
um- Qwashu,		155	i- Yeza le-Illaba,		147
in- Qwebebana,		155	i- Yeza lezi-Kali,		81, 115
i- Qwili,		67	i- Yeza eli-Mnyama,		121
			i- Yeza lo-Moya olubomvu,		90
i- Rau,		82, 113	i- Yeza len-Tshulube,		131
i- Rubuxa,		65, 90	i- Yeza loko-Xaxasisa,		119
i- Savu,		154	in- Zinziniba,		59, 101
ubu-Shwa,		81			

INDEX OF ENGLISH AND DUTCH NAMES OF PLANTS.

Agrimony,	108	Guarri, Bosch, ... 116
Aloe, Medicinal,	120	
Aloe, Small, ..	105	Hemp, ... 28, 164
Aloe, White-spotted,	.. 73, 133	Honde-bos, ... 131
Anemone, ...	121	Horsewood, ... 112
Arum, The common,	76	
Asparagus, ..	183	Kaffir-tree, Small, ... 90
Assegai-wood,	171	Kalmoes, ... 8, 67
		Kalmoes, Berg, ... 67
Bietouw, ..	179	Kanker-bos, .. 62, 66, 86, 116, 138
Bitter apple, ..	130	Knobwood, ... 44, 58
Bitter blar, ..	126, 169	Kruidje roer mij niet, .. 32, 83
Bitter wortel,	61	Kruisbesje, ... 171
Blue-gum, ..	95, 99, 174	
Boter-bloem,	141, 178	Leeuw hout, ... 69
		Lichen, A, ... 41
Cactus, ..	225	Lightning shrub, ... 171
Cancer-bush, ..	62, 66, 116, 138	Lily, The Egyptian, .. 78
Caper-bush, ..	156	Limoen Gras, ... 182
Capive, Wild,	.. 89, 130	Limoen hout, .. 160, 179
Cardamom, Wild,	58	Loog 182
Castor-oil shrub,	123	
Clematis, ..	101, 161	Mallow, The, ... 74
Convolvulus, Larger,	174	Meste kruid, ... 92
Cotton, Wild,	61	Milk-wood, White, ... 155
		Mistletoe, The, ... 176
Dagga, Common,	.. 28, 164	
Dagga, Klip,	.. 20, 25, 29, 155	Nettle, The, ... 113
Dagga, Red, ..	20, 25, 27, 103, 106	Nightshade, The, ... 59, 133
Davidjes, ..	43, 86, 143	Nightshade, Deadly, .. 149
Dock, Smaller,	107	
		Olive, ... 109
Euphorbia, ..	119	Oonth bosje, ... 154
Fern, Hard, ..	102	Paarde praam, .. 44, 58, 126
		Padde klauw, 20, 30, 59, 62, 128
Gall-sick bush, The Albany,	154	Parsley, ... 134
Gift-bol, ..	158, 180	Peach, The, ... 79, 165
Goose-foot, ..	129, 173	Pink, The, ... 147
Goud bloem,	81	Plantain, The, ... 82

Plumbago, The,	..	.. 148	Scabious,	.. ..	.. 113
Poison-bush, Bushman's,		.. 37, 158	Sheep's ear, ..	..	.. 101
Pomegranate,	..	109, 117	Sorrel,	.. ..	.. 107
Prickly pear,	..	.. 225	Stramonium,	..	.. 123
Pumpkin seeds,	..	.. 109	Sweet-potato, Wild,		.. 151
Rabassam or Rabas,		115, 168	Traveller's joy,	..	..101, 161
Ranunculus,..	..	70, 102, 165			
River pumpkin,	..	.. 161	Wait-a-bit, The,	..	.. 88, 136
Rooi houtje,..	..	.. 89, 117	Willow, The Native,		94
Rooi wortel,	..	.. 84, 135	Worldwise, ..	..	.. 148
			Wormwood, ..	..	.. 95, 99
Saffron wood,	..	.. 178	Wormwood, River, ..		.. 58, 147

Printed at the Lovedale Mission Press.

A CONTRIBUTION
TO SOUTH AFRICA MATERIA MEDICA,
BY ANDREW SMITH OF ST. CYRUS, M.A.

Press Notices of previous Edition.

It is with very great pleasure that we have perused the above work. It is not too much to say that we have never seen a book written by a non-professional man that was so valuable a contribution to medical science . . . . . The chapter on snake poison antidotes is exceptionally good. Two species of *Leonotis*, *Teucrium Africanum*, *Melianthus comosus*, *Blepharis Capensis*, *Crabbea cirsioides*, and several others are classed as remedies under this heading. . . We must however resist the temptation to quote further from this most interesting book, which is a veritable "fact heap."—*South African Medical Journal*.

At Lovedale at any rate the importance of medical science as a handmaid to religion receives due recognition. We have long looked for information such as is here presented in manual and very handy form, as to the possible value of the contributions which South Africa can make towards the provision of medicinal drugs. . . . .
. . . The chapters on cobra and viper poisons, remedies for snake-bite, plants as reme lies for stomach an l liver disorders, (and for those) arising from blood-poisoning, will be found of more than technical and professional interest ; while the advice contained in the chapters on lung-sickness, gall-sickness, horse-sickness, and all the ills that cattle-flesh is heir to, will, especially as it is couched in language clear and telling, prove worthy of study by stock farmers. Some able Appendices on consumption among civilized Natives, fruits in relation to climate, redwater, pasture and graminivora, bring a very valuable and interesting contribution to one of the most important branches of scientific investigation. It is in the production of literature such as this that Lovedale will prove an important factor in urging forward the welfare of South Africa generally. —*East London Dispatch*.

This is a work worthy of all attention in scientific circles, while to the general reader, if he have any knowledge of country "house remedies," it will be pleasant to check his his knowledge by what is here set down, as the names of all the South African medical plants known to the author are given in Dutch as well as Kaffir, and the botanical name is also given for scientific identification . . . . The book is beautifully printed and the matter carefully arranged.—*The Argus*.

The Lovedale Institution, at which this valuable work is published, has done most important work for the benefit of the Natives of South Africa, for which all classes must be thankful. Missionaries not only elevate and improve those for whom they leave home and the higher civilization, but they make their pupils capable of advancing the well-being of those Europeans who settle among them, or employ their necessary services. . . . . The work is exceedingly interesting even to a reader without botanical or medical knowledge. The names of plants are given scientifically, and in both Dutch and Kaffir. Many most valuable antidotes to poisons may thus be easily identified by any intelligent and observant person.—*Church News for South Africa*.

That the labour expended in its compilation is evidenced on every page.

That a perusal of its interesting contents will convince even the most casual observer, that our South African *veld* and "bush" abound in priceless medicinal plants.— *Grocott's Mail*.

It adds a fresh interest to one's walks abroad, to be able to recognise very many, if not most, of the plants here named, as growing in our immediate vicinity. Mr. Smith's description of them is quite sufficient for the botanical student. The general reader cannot expect to identify a specimen from the description given ; but should a plant be inquired for under its Native name, and a wrong plant substituted for it, the general reader if careful will usually be able to detect the imposition. We express our high opinion of the work, and recommend all interested to procure it for themselves.—*Bedford Enterprise*.

SHORT PAPERS
CHIEFLY ON SOUTH AFRICAN SUBJECTS.
BY

ANDREW SMITH of St. CYRUS, M.A.

Lovedale: Book Department.

Edinburgh: Andrew Elliot.

(In Cloth, neat, pp. 224, Three shillings, Postage 3½d

PRESS NOTICES.

The scope of these articles is most comprehensive, embracing discussions on almost every department of life, religious, mental, moral, physical, social, and scientific, not even excluding some of the difficult problems of our political condition in relation to the Natives of this country. . . . . It consists of short articles in the main, admirably condensed and very suggestive, affording ample matter for thought, giving arguments in brief, and the conclusions arrived at by a thoughtful and cultured mind. . . . . The Book is well printed, handy in form, which always makes reading pleasant, and it contains that which makes every book of any value more valuable—a good index.—*Eastern Province Herald.*

The book is unique and a most valuable contribution to South African literature. There is nothing in the preface to show whether the author is professor, parson, or doctor. He may be any of these, or all these in one. There is a freshness about his thoughts that ought to make the book a favourite with all classes of readers. . . . . Most cordially do we recommend this book as containing a mass of information clearly stated and vigorously argued. It throws much clear light on the southern portion of the "dark continent."—*Grocott's Mail.*

It is within the range of subjects in their (Native) group that "*Imvo*"—Native Opinion—will find that which affects the saving of its people from mental, moral, social, physical, and political destruction. The Editor of that paper cannot too frequently turn to the points Mr. Smith raises if he will impress the educated Natives with a lively sense of their condition, and how they are to be prevented from improving themselves off the face of the earth. . . . . If for nothing else in the book, we strongly commend this section of it—Native Social Questions—to all our fellow-colonists.—*Cape Mercury.*

The part of it which is likely to prove of special interest and value to them (Teachers) is that which treats of the Intellectual Method in Education. It includes chapters on Natural History and Physical Geography, both treated of in such a manner as to make the reader think and reason out for himself, and to make most readers feel ashamed of their own ignorance in the face of such a breadth of sound and suggestive information . . . . . The reverential spirit in which the series of Bible Studies is conducted will prove impressive even to those who may not agree in all points with the writer. They are lay-sermons of rare value, healthful and manly in tone, as well as kindly and charitable in feeling.—*Educational News.*

He (the Author) writes 'Short Papers' in which he comes at once to the subjects of discussion, and from which he cuts away all useless padding. The result is that he presents his views in clear and terse language. The reader may not be able to accept all his positions, but those who know aught of the tendency of modern economic thought, will be ready to welcome the book as one in which the spirit, if not the phraseology, of the newer schools, manifests itself consciously or unconsciously. But the new Spirit is the old influence of Christian morality, that alone can preserve society, and sweeten the relations that men bear to men.—*Fort Beaufort Advocate.*

www.ingramcontent.com/pod-product-compliance
Lightning Source LLC
Chambersburg PA
CBHW020802230426
43666CB00007B/823